HEAL UP!

For Hannah,

In great health,

Dr. *[signature]*

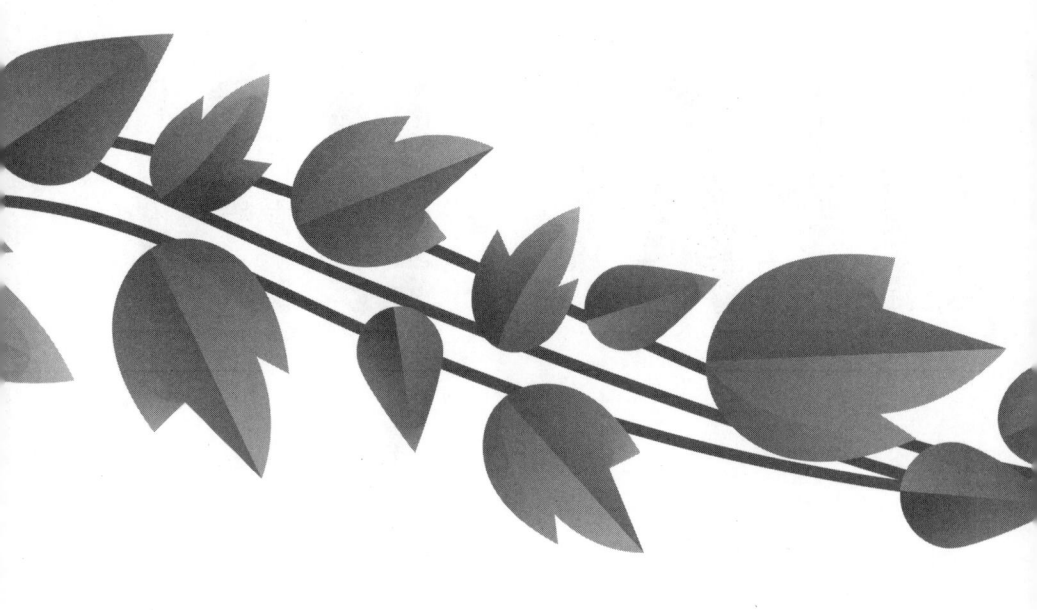

HEAL UP!

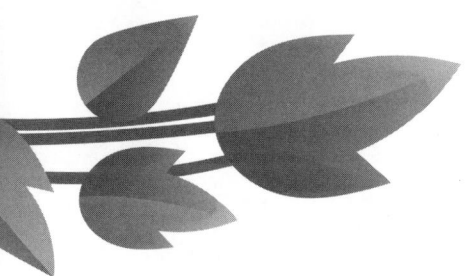

-------- SEVEN WAYS TO --------
FASTER HEALING AND OPTIMUM HEALTH

Dr. Sanda Moldovan

Advantage®

Published by Advantage, Charleston, South Carolina.
Member of Advantage Media Group.

ADVANTAGE is a registered trademark, and the Advantage colophon is a trademark of Advantage Media Group, Inc.

Printed in the United States of America.

10 9 8 7 6 5 4 3 2

ISBN: 978-1-59932-867-6
LCCN: 2018937918

Cover design by Katie Biondo.
Layout design by George Stevens.

This publication is designed to provide accurate and authoritative information in regard to the subject matter covered. It is sold with the understanding that the publisher is not engaged in rendering legal, accounting, or other professional services. If legal advice or other expert assistance is required, the services of a competent professional person should be sought.

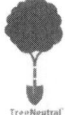
Advantage Media Group is proud to be a part of the Tree Neutral® program. Tree Neutral offsets the number of trees consumed in the production and printing of this book by taking proactive steps such as planting trees in direct proportion to the number of trees used to print books. To learn more about Tree Neutral, please visit **www.treeneutral.com**.

TreeNeutral

Advantage Media Group is a publisher of business, self-improvement, and professional development books and online learning. We help entrepreneurs, business leaders, and professionals share their Stories, Passion, and Knowledge to help others Learn & Grow. Do you have a manuscript or book idea that you would like us to consider for publishing? Please visit **advantagefamily.com** or call **1.866.775.1696**.

To my grandparents, Eleonora and Gavril, for teaching me how to connect to Mother Earth and live in harmony with nature.

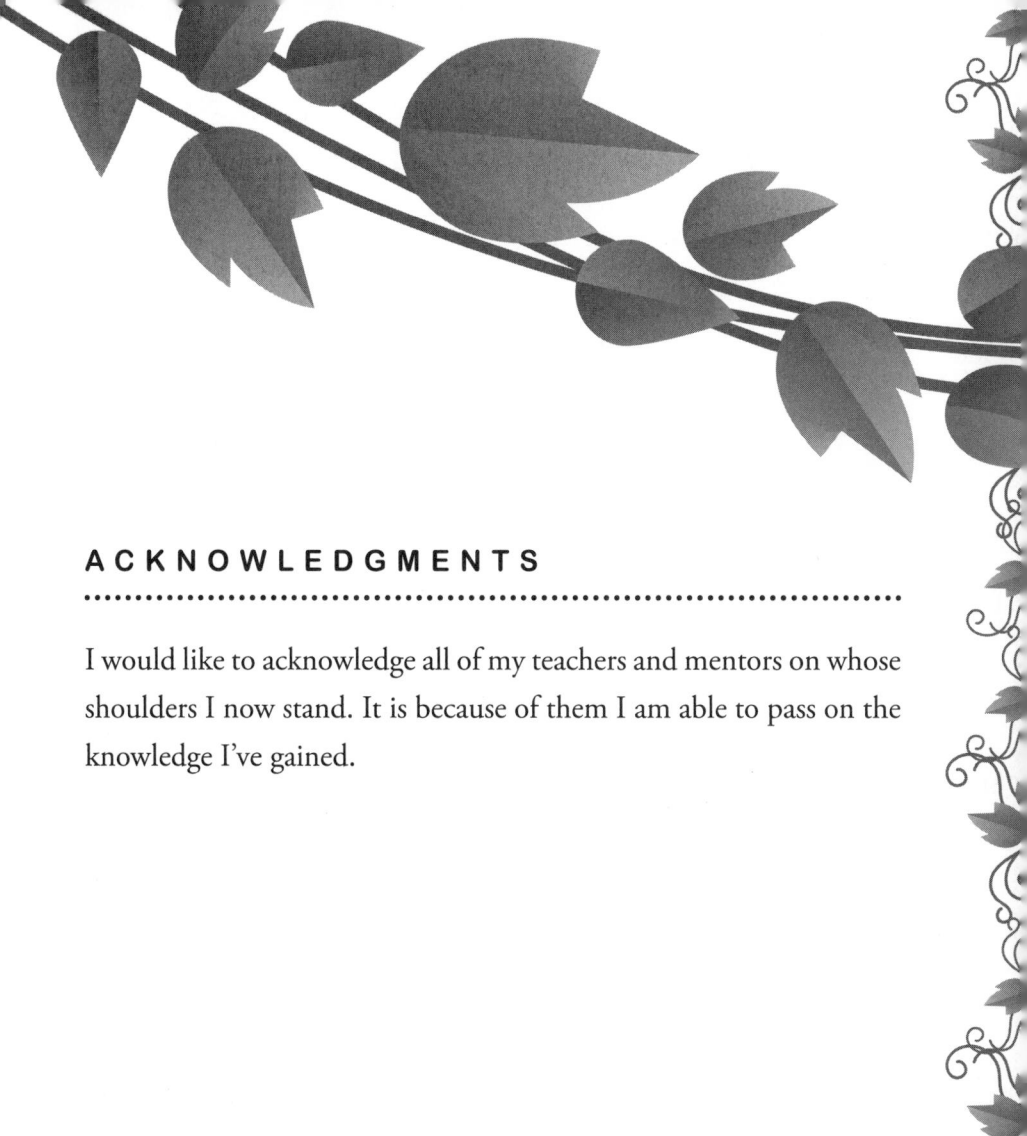

ACKNOWLEDGMENTS

I would like to acknowledge all of my teachers and mentors on whose shoulders I now stand. It is because of them I am able to pass on the knowledge I've gained.

TABLE OF CONTENTS

....

FOREWORD xi

INTRODUCTION 1

CHAPTER 1 7

TODAY'S PROBLEM WITH HEALING

CHAPTER 2 17

HEALING WITH FOOD

CHAPTER 3 55

HEALING WITH LIGHT AND ENERGY

CHAPTER 4 77

HEALING WITH MEDITATION, GUIDED IMAGERY, AND SLEEP

CHAPTER 5 91

HEALING WITH OXYGEN

CHAPTER 6 109

HEALING WITH PLANTS, HERBS, AND TEAS

CHAPTER 7 129

HEALING WITH VITAMINS AND SUPPLEMENTS

CHAPTER 8 161

HEALING WITH WATER

CONCLUSION 175

Recipes for Healing 177
References 187
Our Services 199
About the Author 201

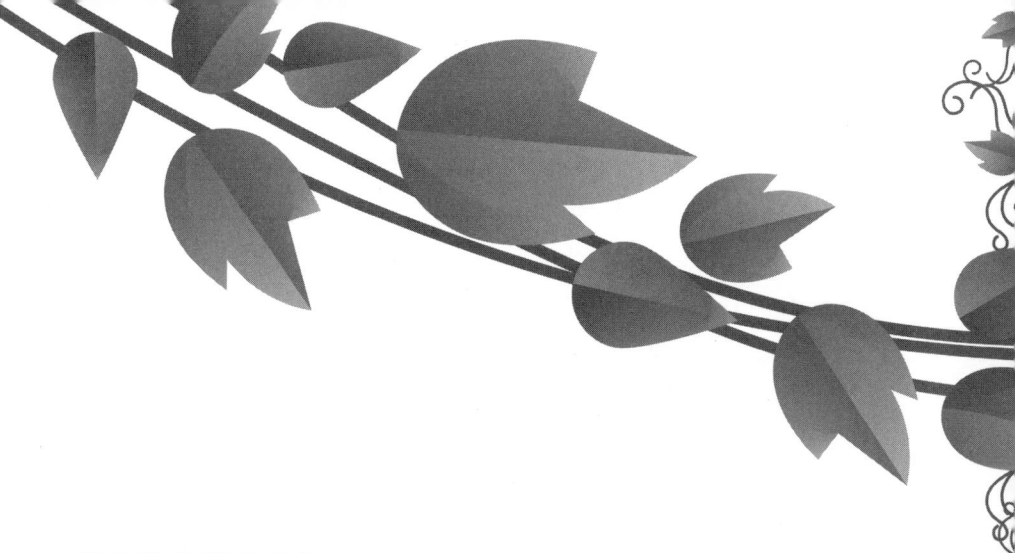

FOREWORD

....

Enthusiastic, inquisitive, passionate, focused, and disciplined. These are the words which describe my impressions of Dr. Sanda Moldovan during the time that she was my student at the UCLA Implant Center fifteen years ago. These first imprints of her willingness to push her knowledge beyond her post-graduate specialty program have never left my mind's eye. They are still truthful representations of who she is today as a leading wellness practitioner.

For almost three decades, I have taught implant dentistry all over the world and proudly witnessed many students excel in life. Sanda is one of my alumnae that has achieved a distinctive edge that elevates her to a lane all her own as a preventative oral health expert.

Her master's degree in oral biology provides the academic foundation for her boundless curiosity about the linkage between inflammation in the mouth and the presence of harmful pathogens in the rest of the body, which can cause inflammation and infections leading to heart disease, endocarditis, cancer, diabetes, HIV/AIDS, and osteoporosis.

Yet, dental professionals do not consistently recognize how reducing inflammation in the mouth is essential for accelerated healing and continued overall health. Sanda treats the slightest oral inflammation with precise care, arresting it before it travels to the rest of the body and is slow to write a plethora of prescriptions for pain and infections when the symptoms can be alleviated with natural supplements, dietary changes, and other therapies.

Sanda's appreciation for the biological responses within the body and its ability to heal has grown, as she is fascinated with its optimal functioning capacities for performance, and feeling and looking better. It's impressive to me how Sanda stays on top of cutting-edge technological advancements and attends numerous health conferences throughout the year to continue her medical and dental education and to provide her patients and her colleagues with the latest knowledge. The demand for her lectures about the importance of connecting the mouth to the rest of the body is steadily attracting interest from more dentists around the globe.

Putting our patients first should be the golden rule for medical and dental practitioners, but sadly, it is not always the case. Sanda is a shining example of how treating people's health issues are about the quality of care, not numbers. She's a successful periodontist and practice owner, yet she never loses sight of the most important component—the patient. She's a very caring person when it comes to them. She treats every individual patient as if he or she is the only one she knows at that moment.

Sanda's ability to translate complex science into understandable and practical terms for her readers is what makes this book an enlightening and enjoyable read. Sanda's authenticity and genuine concern over helping everyone on the planet to live a better life leaps off these pages. She provides relatable, simple, inexpensive, effective, and non-toxic things we can do to maintain good health. By reducing stress and eliminating harmful chemicals from our systems, we can feel refreshed and renewed.

From her years of knowledge and experience, you will be helped with making choices that will drastically improve how you feel each day. Sanda practices what she teaches, as she has acted as her own lab experiment for *Heal Up!* and has incorporated all of the principles and methods contained in this book to her own life. She can share, with unparalleled authority, how you can nurture and nourish the living cells within you.

You are about to embark on a fascinating health journey with an empathetic and caring kindred spirit.

Sascha A. Jovanovic, DDS, MS

Academic Chair of the gIDE Institute

Assistant Professor, Loma Linda University Dental Implant Center

Past-President, European Association for Osseointegration (EAO)

Summer, 2018

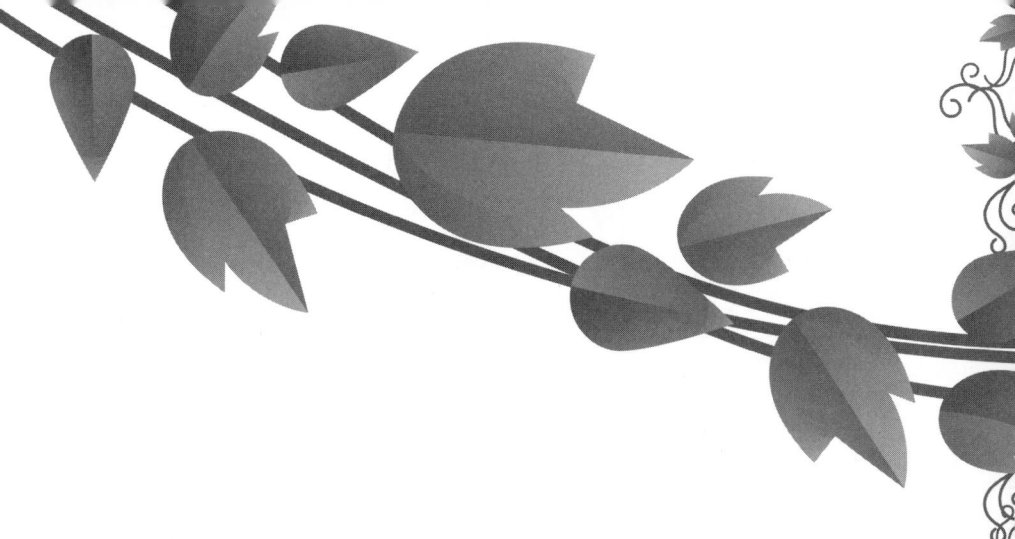

INTRODUCTION

∙∙

I t's interesting how the sum total of my personal and professional experiences ultimately brought me to this exact moment where you and I, maybe total strangers, would meet. Allowing me to share what I know about fulfilling our common desire for preserving our precious health. It's an honor to pass along to you what I have learned from my years as a periodontist about how to treat our bodies with natural remedies before and after surgery.

In this book, you will learn how to reduce recovery time by preventing toxic medications from entering your system so you can heal more efficiently. Prescription medications have their place; however, discovering and using natural alternatives whenever possible prevents potential narcotics abuse and lessens the likelihood of unwelcome side effects. In addition, the cornucopia of non-pharmaceutical wellness aids and treatments are less expensive than conventional medicines, with many of these practical solutions freely available to all of us and supported by our planet's ecosystem. Dr. Mother Nature is the best prescriber and helps with not only healing, but also supporting and ensuring we attain optimum wellness throughout our lives.

Growing up in Communist Romania, I never imagined I would one day enjoy the freedom and privilege of writing a book, where I could share these important truths about authentic healing practices, combined with recent science on nutrition and healing. Where I grew up in Sibiu, Transylvania, there was no free press, so a book about the empowerment of wellness for our bodies, minds, and souls was inconceivable. Yet, that same oppressive regime required my attention to certain eating disciplines which have been proven healthy to this day. My upbringing nurtured my innate curiosity and made me an apprentice to everything you will find of value within the pages that lie ahead.

Today, we take for granted the convenience of having grocery stores packed with shelves full of delectable items to eat, 24/7. But as a child, I can remember aisle after aisle of empty supermarket shelves. My parents had to stand in line for milk or any kind of meat, so if you didn't go early enough in the day, you couldn't even find bananas or apples, even bread wasn't available in the afternoon. You had to have underground connections, or win favor with somebody high up the food chain, if you will, to get many items. For this reason, my parents and every single Romanian family were obligated to store food, to can, to grow our own vegetables, and even raise our own chickens (though we lived in the middle of the city, and both my mom and dad were educated professionals, not farmers by trade). That's the essence of communism—everybody lives as one giant middle class. There is no designated rich vs. poor clashing of classes. A doctor lives the life of a farmer. It's up to your own ingenuity and resourcefulness to eat and live well.

We had a small farm in the back of our house, where we raised poultry. I used to race to help my grandparents clean out the chicken coop where I would fish for eggs. I loved to count them. We even had a couple of little pigs that we butchered for sausages and bacon. My grandparents had a separate house on the same property, as it's customary in Romania for families to live close together. Every day while my parents were at work, my grandmother, Eleanor, taught me about planting and growing vegetables and fruit. Her design for living was rooted in the importance of nurturing a soil that is *alive* and retrieving probiotics from our food and natural minerals. We were composting in the '70s and '80s. Our scraps were put back into the soil to give nutrients back to the vegetables and fruits that we grew, such as tomatoes, cherries, peaches, pears, and apples. Then we canned. Nothing was wasted.

My mom and grandmother pressurized and sterilized jars to preserve spring, summer and autumn foods—whatever we cultivated would be what we had for the winter. As a result, we had plenty of good meats, vegetables, and fruits which lasted us until the end of winter. Our daily menu always consisted of meat and fermented vegetables, which were raw and filled with natural probiotics, decades before they were in vogue, as they are today. Not canned with citric acid. We used to pick wild mushrooms in the Romanian forests after a rainfall. I so enjoyed searching for the green leaves and finding the chanterelles. Little did I know that I would one day recommend mushrooms for their anti-cancer therapeutics to my nutrition clients. It was years later that science proved organic foods have more nutrition than conventionally grown foods, and how dangerous pesticides are for our health. In the United States, we are now going back to these basic ways of growing and harvesting our food as we step away from the processed foods in the stores which contribute to inflammation and poor healing. Usually, our selection was cabbage or carrots, and various greens, but you can pickle cauliflower, peppers, anything that's vegetarian. I learned the importance of feeding my digestive tract fermented foods, which is consistently lacking in today's Western civilization. It is why I believe we see so many GI (Gastrointestinal) problems. Probiotics are necessary for the healing of ulcers, periodontal disease, the gut, and the brain.

Being grounded in the earth is extremely important. The moment Ol' Man Winter was saying goodbye, we were packing picnics and eating outside. We would find a patch of green grass and lay out our meal for the day on a cloth. My brother John and I would run barefoot in the grass. No wonder we were so happy—as science tells us that connecting our bare feet to the ground negatively charges us to be in greater harmony with planet Earth. This has a positive effect on our thoughts, moods, and anxiety levels. As they were deeply religious, my grandparents also required we pray together for a good ten minutes each evening, which later morphed into meditation practices consisting of a wealth of methods I have exposed myself to over the years. Whether it was digging in the cool earth planting crops, oil-painting alongside my grandmother from the still life of the many God-given scenes around us, or even changing a car's spark plugs under the tutelage of my mechanical engineer dad who could fix anything, I was always working with my hands.

I'm convinced my eventual careers were chosen for me as a result of the hobbies and interests greatly influenced by my parents and grandparents. For instance, my grandfather, Gavril, was a physics and math professor. As a fourteen-year-old, there were many times where I sat with him as he read from magazines about problem solving and much of what I now know to be classified as quantum physics. Sure enough, today I am talking quantum physics. Even then, I grasped how we are all comprised of energy; how outside energy sources can influence our cellular health; how our teeth are alive, growing inside our jawbones. My fascination with energy treating devices and non-invasive lasers has led me to acquire the latest in technological advances for my practice, which is of such great value to my patients—but often draws a stern look of disapproval from my CPA upon my return from a technology conference, where I've ordered more equipment.

As my father, John, taught me every use known to man for a screwdriver, dental implants just come down to knowing how to drill a hole with a screwdriver. Dental implants are actually biomechanical devices that insert into the jawbone to replace missing teeth. A few years ago, when I performed surgery on my dad to replace his missing teeth with implants, he looked at my drills, and said, "I think I can help you design these better."

I believe another reason I majored in biology in college was due to watching my mother, also named Sanda, test precious metals at the National Bank of Romania. As a chemical engineer, she was responsible for employing various solutions to test the gems and metals to verify their authenticity. She would explain the process of achieving the results when I would visit her working.

So, despite the disadvantages of living under a dictatorship, I was blessed to have an education that is priceless. I became an expert in natural healing at an early age and learned to respect and value our planet's most essential and prized gift: our individual health. We are all creatures of this universe with fundamental laws for our basic needs. When we ignore or violate these laws is when we get into trouble, and our overall health suffers. It doesn't have to cost the world to maintain a healthy lifestyle. You don't have to be rich to go for a walk in a park or barefoot along a beach. You just have to be willing to take action and control of your well being.

This is your book. I wrote it for you. My motivation was the hope that it educates and inspires you to pick yourself up wherever you are on your journey toward greater health as well as excite you to keep moving forward. As you know, we only get one body, one mind, one soul.

If you are one of the millions of people who are suffering from pain, fatigue, or healing slowly from an injury, then the practical applications of this book's contents will undoubtedly change your life! The chapters are not intended to be read in any particular order. Start with the one that mostly calls out to you. Every step in this book will contribute to healing. All you need is the willingness and an open mind and heart.

In great health,

Dr. Sanda Moldovan

Beverly Hills, California

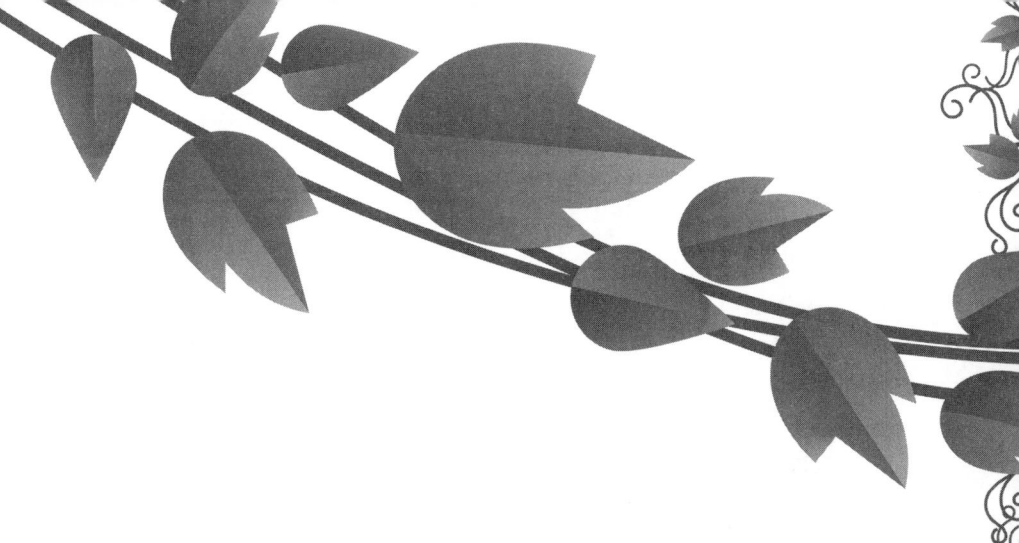

....

CHAPTER 1

TODAY'S PROBLEM WITH HEALING

R ecently, at lunchtime, I was in the elevator of the medical building at the University of California, Los Angeles. Next to me were two nurses carrying their lunch trays loaded with fried chicken and mac and cheese—and let's not forget the white bread.

On their trays was what is known as the Standard American Diet (SAD), which is far from a healthy diet. Yet that is what's being served in hospitals for health professionals and patients. I cringed and thought: Where are the nutrients? I wanted so desperately to reach out and add some rainbow colors to their plates for antioxidants and phytonutrients.

We are facing an epidemic of chronic inflammation, not only in United States, but globally. Chronic inflammation can manifest in many ways: cardiovascular disease, obesity, diabetes, high cholesterol, rheumatoid arthritis or periodontitis, cavities, and oral ulcers, to name a few. How can we improve or accelerate healing from a small wound, such as a wisdom tooth removal or even chronic disease? In this book you will discover several different ways to implement at-home techniques to take your healing potential to a higher level.

Just as the eyes are windows to the soul, the mouth is the gateway to a person's health and well-being.

• • • • • • • • • • • • • • • •

Microscopic injuries happen every day. Our bodies repair and heal different areas every day. When we eat crunchy foods, we injure our mouth, typically on a daily basis, and most of the time we don't even notice. We heal. Healing happens daily, therefore daily support of our cells and immune system is a must.

As a periodontist, I know that inflammation of the gums or ulcerations in the mouth are indicative of someone's overall health. Just as the eyes are windows to the soul, *the mouth is the gateway to a person's health and well-being.* As a nutritionist, I correlate oral problems and diseases, like cavities, aphthous ulcers, and gum disease to overall nutritional deficiencies. In this book, I will show you how to stay nutritionally fit to heal faster and prevent any future manifestations of oral diseases.

BEHIND THE EPIDEMIC

When a person incurs an injury, whether during a sports activity, surgery, or invasion by bacteria or a virus, the body's first response is to become inflamed. According to Stedman's Medical Dictionary, inflammation is a localized protective reaction of tissue to irritation, injury, or infection characterized by pain, redness, swelling, and sometimes loss of function.

Inflammation is the first stage in the healing process, occurring when the body's cells rush at the site of injury to start the repair process. A normal, acute inflammatory response involving heat, pain, swelling, and redness typically follow an injury or surgery of an organ, tissues, bones, and joints, lasting several days. The inflammatory stage is necessary for good healing; however, inflammation that does not subside after a few days and continues for more than a week is considered to be chronic.

Chronic inflammation sets the stage for continuous or intermittent pain and swelling, as well as possible autoimmune diseases. Chronic inflammation occurs because the immune system is overactivated and fails to turn off, perceiving a constant, foreign attack on the body.

Where is this chronic inflammation epidemic coming from? Mainly, the Standard American Diet 's lack of nutrients combined with today's fast-paced lifestyles, which can cause an accumulation of toxins and stress in the body.

At my practice, Beverly Hills Dental Health and Wellness, we treat the patient as a whole. As a periodontist and nutritionist, I know that when a person has oral health problems, most of the time, it is correlated to another health issue. We believe the mouth is the gateway to health. What does that mean? It means the mouth tells a story of the past. Everything a person experiences—air, water, food, stress, depression—leaves its mark on their body. For instance, cavities are a result of bad eating habits, and tooth wear from grinding is a result of stress. Teeth are little organs, capable of healing from cavities and disease.

Our team of dentists and health care practitioners sees patients who are often not nutritionally fit. We have a world epidemic of people who are overfed and undernourished, and those conditions wreak havoc on their bodies—physically and mentally. The problem can become an endless and debilitating cycle. For instance, seasonal affective disorder can lead to depression. If a person is depressed, they probably do not care enough to brush their teeth, much less visit the dentist. This creates more problems inside the mouth, which can make it more difficult to eat healthy foods. Without addressing the root cause—inadequate nutrition leading to chronic inflammation—the person's health problems will continue to escalate. It's a vicious cycle in need of help from a team of health care professionals.

Most chronic inflammation starts in the gastro-intestinal tract. Some 70 percent of the immune system lines the intestines. When partially digested food particles leak into the bloodstream, the immune system is activated because these food particles are seen as "invaders." Only the nutrients from food belong in the bloodstream. It has been shown that this "leaky gut" issue can start in infancy, it goes undetected and then leads to systemic inflammatory response syndrome (SIRS), inflammatory bowel disease, type 1 diabetes, allergies, asthma, and autism. With "leaky guts" we also see "leaky gums," as the mouth is the opening of the gastrointestinal tract. How can this be healed? It comes back to diet, eliminating harmful foods, and adding good bacteria/probiotics.

In chronic inflammation, immune complexes—composed of immune cells, bacteria, and toxins—circulate throughout the body. Most are eliminated through the liver, but, if there are too many, then the liver is overwhelmed and the complexes start accumulating in the tissues. Some researchers have shown that nutritional deficiencies in trace minerals have contributed to the inability of the liver to cope with and discard these immune complexes. How do we facilitate the healing of the liver to cope with these issues? It comes back to food and rest.

Sometimes years of chronic inflammation set in before symptoms manifest themselves. For example, with heart disease (the number one killer of women in the United States) years of chronic inflammation of the arteries likely occur before any chest pains arise. There is also increasing epidemiologic evidence for a positive association between periodontal disease and cardiovascular disease, both with an inflammatory component. Many diseases have chronic inflammation as a precursor: Alzheimer's, cancer, Parkinson's, autoimmune diseases (celiac disease, Lupus and multiple sclerosis), oral diseases such as periodontitis and oral ulcers. As dentists, we can see the inflammation in the mouth way before the heart shows symptoms. And let's not forget about the microbiome, which makes up all the microorganisms covering our bodies inside and out, including the mouth. As a periodontist, I treat and analyze the oral bacteria and other pathogens. Dr. David Perlmutter, in his book *Brain Maker*, describes the microbiome as the key to human health. He presents research for a strong connection between the gut bacteria and the brain, the immune system, mood, and metabolism.

CAUSES OF CHRONIC INFLAMMATION

- **Leaky gut**
- **Food sensitivities**
- **Toxin accumulation**
- **Ongoing stress**
- **Sugar in excess**
- **Obesity**
- **Smoking**
- **Lack of sleep**

Eliminating toxins, maintaining proper oral hygiene, eating healthy, drinking plenty of water, and calming the mind are a few ways to combat chronic inflammation and promote a healthy microbiome. As a periodontist, I focus on preventing oral diseases and recovering properly from a surgical procedure or condition; that is the central point of this book. True healing can only be achieved by overcoming chronic inflammation.

While chronic inflammation is detrimental to healing, inflammation that occurs following an incision or injury is essential for proper healing. Also known as acute inflammation, the inflammation that occurs during healing is one of three stages: stage 1 is when blood clots form; stage 2 is when swelling and helpful inflammation occurs; stage 3 is when tissue repairs and rebuilds.

WHAT CAN YOU GAIN FROM THIS BOOK?

The following factors are critical in achieving health. These can also factor into your ability to heal and to repair, rebuild, and renew naturally.

Diet. A healthy diet is crucial to healing. How much sugar do you use? How much processed food do you consume? How much alcohol do you drink? How many servings of vegetables and fruits do you eat a day? All of these can impact how well your body heals.

Exercise. According to the CDC Guidelines, adults should get at least 150 minutes a week of aerobic exercise, and two or more days of muscle strengthening activity. For those over sixty-five, this activity should be increased. Less than 50 percent of adults get adequate aerobic activity and only 20 percent meet the requirements for both aerobic and muscle-strengthening activity. Exercise helps your heart and circulation. It also reduces stress and oxygenates your brain and body. People who are physically fit tend to have less pain and recover faster.

Stress. When we have ongoing stress at home or at work, we don't heal well. It is important to find coping skills first to learn to relax, such as hobbies, meditation, or yoga. The three most stressful events in a person's life are a death in the family, moving, and divorce. Avoid any medical surgical procedures if any of these have occurred recently. Give yourself time to heal emotionally first.

Sleep. A lack of sleep can also affect recovery. If sleep continues to elude you, consider acupuncture and guided meditation techniques to help you get the much-needed rest we need. Hormonal balance is also an important factor to being able to sleep properly.

Weight. Excess weight increases the risk for chronic inflammation, diabetes, and slower healing. More than one-third of Americans are overweight and close to 40 percent are obese. A body-mass index (BMI) of between 25 and 29.9 is considered overweight; above that is obese. Use the BMI table from The National Institute of Health to determine your BMI. If you are struggling to lose weight, you are not alone. A support group such as foodaddicts.org might help. Food addiction is very real and it is important to find the right support group.

Smoking. More than 480,000 Americans die annually as a consequence of smoking. Studies show that smokers who have had medical or dental surgery heal 10-20 percent slower than non-smokers, and the complication rates are higher. Quitting can increase the success of recovering from surgery or an injury.

Genomics. Genome sequencing has provided us with new insights into healing. Today, a person's entire genome can be mapped out from a strand of hair for just a couple of hundred dollars. Some genome information still remains a mystery, but some of it has proven to be very valuable, revealing that certain gene sequences are related to more inflammation, breast cancer, or heart disease.[1] It shows us how we individually process foods. Where an additional cup of coffee, although detrimental to the heart for some, it is beneficial for others, to give an example. It can also reveal how we metabolize different pain medications for those suffering from chronic pain.

AN OPPORTUNITY FOR NATURAL HEALING

Health professionals have an amazing opportunity today: We can make our communities healthier by encouraging patients to adopt a healthier lifestyle. Statistics show that more people go to the dentist for a check-up than to their physician for a physical. By incorporating a short nutritional survey into the consultation, we encourage patients to make lifestyle changes that will improve not only their oral health, but also their overall health.

Yet, in spite of all that is known about nutrition's impact on inflammation and healing, healthy eating is rarely a part of the discussion when a patient visits a doctor or a dentist. In fact, a recent poll shows that only 4 percent of dental practices offer any form of nutritional counseling.

As a periodontist and nutritionist, I frequently meet dentists from all over the world. I know that most dental offices don't have a nutritional questionnaire. Other than brushing and flossing, most dentists don't ask a patient about their health habits, even though those habits are key to a person's oral health and overall wellness.

---

1   For example, the genetic sequence of the enzyme responsible for folic acid use is called MTHFR. Some 30 percent of people have a genetic deficiency that prevents their body from absorbing folic acid or making it usable in their body. These people are more prone to inflammation, poor healing, and cardiovascular problems. A simple saliva test can show if this genetic variation is present, and when identified, it can be easily repaired by supplementation with the methylated version of folic acid.

That questionnaire should ask about their nutritional and other health practices, as well as ask about the patient's dietary supplements, as these can cause blood thinning or interaction with some medications, causing other health problems.

TABLE 1: NUTRITIONAL SURVEY FOR THE DENTAL PRACTICE

Are you currently taking nutritional supplements?			Yes	No
Multivitamin	Vitamin D	Fish Oils	Herbal	Homeopathic
List all other supplements:				
Are any of these prescribed by a nutritionist or doctor?			Yes	No
If yes, list the name and phone number:				
Are you on a special diet?				
Vegan	Vegetarian		Gluten-free	Other:
Do you experience any of the following:				
Loss of appetite	Fatigue		Constipation	Diarrhea
Muscle cramping	Bruising		Digestive problems	Hair loss
Slow wound healing	Sleeplessness		Skin conditions	Nausea
Vitamin D level (if known):				

Having a successful dental practice is about creating long-lasting relationships with patients—treating the whole, not the hole in their mouth. Some of my patients have benefited more from one piece of my nutritional advice than any dental procedure I performed.

For instance, some report that probiotics are now part of their daily regimen, or that their canker sores indicate gluten intolerance. Some tell their friends about the advice I have shared, which adds to the tremendous satisfaction and joy I get from helping them.

Having seen so many afflictions from poor attention to healing, I put together this book to help everyone gain insights into natural options for improving health in order to reduce inflammation and promote healing.

CHAPTER 2
....

HEALING WITH FOOD

T he father of medicine, Hippocrates, identified food as the single universal nutrient needed to promote health. He believed that "all diseases begin in the stomach."

I learned the hard way that "you are what you eat" when I went through my own transformation and healing through food. In my late twenties, I suffered from hypoglycemia, which led me to believe I needed a regular dose of sugar every few hours, so I wouldn't feel fatigued. Fortunately, after recognizing my plight, my neighbor at the time introduced me to the concept of proper nutrition. The first nutrition book I read was by Dr. Gabriel Cousens, called *Conscious Eating*. It helped wean me off my sugar addiction with low-glycemic sugar substitutes.

That is what first led me on the path of exploring the role of food in the body. Just what is that role? Food makes us happy, gives us more energy, speeds up healing, and can keep the body healthy by ridding it of toxins. The bottom line is that food is nourishment. Its role is to fuel our everyday thoughts and physical activities. Food is information for our genes.

However, upon closer scrutiny, food may not be all it seems. Some of that "nourishment" we consume may actually be causing more harm than originally thought. In fact, in the last five years, over seventeen thousand articles published in medical journals have related nutritional deficiency to high blood pressure, diabetes, immune problems, pain, fibromyalgia, and even cancer.

Good nutrition is especially important to the healing process. There are a number of ways for a person with sub-optimal health, and/or someone who's healing after surgery or injury, to improve their condition through better nutrition.

PERSONALIZED NUTRITION

Today, there is a movement toward personalized medicine and nutrition to restore health. Proven over and over again through the fields of epigenetics and nutrigenomics, every single one of us has a different genetic makeup. There's no one-size-fits-all nutritional advice anymore. Each person has a different way of absorbing and processing vitamins and minerals, so not everyone should be taking the same dose of nutrients.

An individual's nutritional requirements are based on their genetics, age, level of activity, intestinal absorption, transport and storage of nutrients. That level of variability is one reason why it is very difficult to isolate a single nutrient in a human study. Compounding the problem is that vitamins and minerals work together—one cannot perform the function without the other, and they cannot be separated for individual study.

Nutritional deficiencies manifest in the mouth. Redness at the corners of the mouth, a shiny, spotted or glossy tongue, a burning mouth, or bleeding gums, can all be signs of different vitamin and nutrient deficiencies. Similarly, ulcers on the tongue or cheek may indicate food intolerance. I am not a fan of prescribing corticosteroids to mask the problem. Instead, we should get to the root of it.

The best way to find out an individual's nutritional status today is via blood testing. Although blood tests are viable tools for making nutritional recommendations, nutritionists rarely rely solely on them.

An individual's nutritional requirements are based on their genetics, age, level of activity, intestinal absorption, transport and storage of nutrients.

. . . .

A test for micronutrients was developed by William Shive, PhD, who realized the importance of identifying which factors limit the nutritional response of each patient. His company, SpectraCell Laboratories, tests cells' behavior in solutions that lack a specific nutrient. The test currently looks for a full range of vitamins, minerals, and other nutrients. The results of the test reveal food groups that will replenish a specific nutrient deficiency, making it easy for the practitioner to give a recommendation.

While the test is comprehensive, it does not include many more nutrients involved in health and healing. But there is ongoing and abundant research in the field of micronutrient testing, and new information comes out constantly.

A food diary is another necessary tool to help determine a person's response to the foods they are eating. A food diary can create a foundation for determining the best nutrition catered to your needs. However, your dietary needs may change over time, and may be impacted by activity level, stressors (including pregnancy), age, or whether you are in a healing process.[2]

FOOD DIARY

	Food	Drink	Sugar
Breakfast			
Snack			
Lunch			
Snack			
Dinner			

Food is information, and what the body does with that information varies from person to person. Some people may digest protein better than others; some survive better on a higher-carbohydrate diet. Some people bloat when consuming bread or pasta, and must consider whether gluten-free is the best option for them. In short, there is no one-size-fits-all diet. What you eat may trigger specific responses in

---

2   In using the word "dietary" or "diet," I am not referring to some sort of short-term restrictions to lose weight. I am simply referring to what you consume on a daily basis.

your genes, and when you understand those responses, you can live healthier and heal faster.

I believe that we should get most of our nutrients from diet first before turning to supplements. As Hippocrates once said, "Let food be thy medicine and medicine be thy food." That statement still holds true today. Unfortunately, most people do not get the necessary nutrients from their food. Statistics from SpectraCell Laboratories show that 70 percent of people tested were deficient in multiple nutrients, including subjects who were already taking supplements.

NUTRITION DURING HEALING

Since there are multiple nutrients involved in healing, only a few of today's health care practitioners incorporate nutrition as part of their recovery protocol.

The requirements for soft tissue healing vs. bone healing vary slightly, but one thing they both have in common is the need for antioxidants. To explain the significance of antioxidants in healing, let me first explain how surgery and injury raise the level of oxidative stress. Oxidative stress essentially refers to the balance of free radicals (essentially harmful cells) and antioxidants in the body. The human body produces free radicals every day as a byproduct of regular cell functions. Free radicals can also be produced by exposure to pollution, poor diet, and certain medications. After an injury or surgery, more free radicals are produced as part of the repair process in healing.

To combat the potential damage done by free radicals, a healing body needs proper levels of antioxidants, which can be increased by consuming the proper foods. Since cooking destroys most anti-oxidants, fresh fruits and vegetables are one of the best sources for people to consume. Basically, the more colorful the foods, the more antioxidants they have. Green, leafy vegetables also contain a healthy supply of minerals and chlorophyll, both of which aid in the rehabilitation process. The intake of chlorophyll can even help with body odor and improve bad breath. When it comes to bone healing, for instance following a fracture, fissure, or dental implant, more minerals are required. Bone healing is typically associated with calcium, but several other essential minerals are also needed, including magnesium, phosphorus, copper, and zinc.

Main nutrients involved in soft tissue healing	Main nutrients involved in bone regeneration
Vitamins: A, Bs, C, E, K, P	Vitamins A, C, D, K
Biotin, copper, chromium, sulphur	Calcium, magnesium, copper, zinc
Essential fatty acids, essential amino acids	Trace minerals, phosphorus, boron

Wound healing in general requires a higher level of proteins, as well as sufficient amounts of carbohydrates and fats. Unfortunately, hospital food following surgery—even oral surgery—often lacks good nutrition. In the first few weeks following major surgery, the requirement for protein may double; as a general rule, dosage should include one gram of protein per pound of body weight.

Diets low in protein, as well as high in sugar and animal fat, can increase inflammation and delay healing. Consuming too much animal fat and hydrogenated vegetable fats, such as margarine, are commonly found in processed foods and may also cause excessive inflammation. But do not eliminate fats completely from the diet. Instead, healthy fats—such as olives, flax seed, nuts and seeds, avocado, coconut oil, and even in raw butter from grass-fed animals—should be added to the diet. Diets rich in omega-3 fatty acids, found in cold-water fish, like salmon and black cod, have been shown to decrease pain and inflammation. Good fats are also necessary for skin to retain its elasticity.

Collagen (a type of protein that appears as ropes under the skin) is also important to healing; connective tissue and bone require collagen formation in order to repair. Collagen production decreases with age, which is why the body begins to wrinkle and is more prone to osteoporosis. Foods rich in vitamin C, such as strawberries and dark green vegetables like brussel sprouts and kale, are necessary for good collagen production. Other foods that aid collagen include beans and starchy root vegetables, like potatoes and sweet potatoes, which help produce hyaluronic acid—an essential part of the connective tissue onto which the collagen fibers form. Foods rich in sulphur, such as olives, arugula, celery; those rich in vitamin A, such as carrots and sweet potatoes; and soy products, which contain an ingredient called genistein, all give collagen an extra boost.

THE BASICS OF WOUND HEALING

Whatever the cause of the wound, there are essentially four stages to its healing.

Stage 1: Blood Clot Formation. Within the first twenty-four hours following any incision, cuts, or scrapes, your body's first priority is to stop the bleeding. Specialized cells from within the blood vessels, called platelets, lay down the glue-like substance that forms the blood clot. This acts as a scaffold for cells to come in and repair the site.

Stage 2: Inflammation. Within two to five days of the event, swelling will occur—usually the second day following the event is the worst. Blood vessels dilate and cells are called to the site to clean out any bacteria or debris. The area will turn red and be warmer to the touch. Although the activity is often mistaken for infection, it is all a normal part of healing. Taking prescription or over-the-counter pain medication to suppress inflammation can slow the healing, so it is advisable to take it only if absolutely necessary. Instead, some good alternatives for pain include enzymes, microcurrent therapy using low-level electric currents, or homeopathy, which is medicine based on the idea that the body can heal itself. In the chapters ahead I will discuss multiple ways to improve the body's ability to repair, rebuild, and renew naturally with food; light and energy; mediation; guided imagery; sleep; oxygen; plants, herbs, and teas; supplements; and water.

Stage 3: Repair and Rebuild. Although the repair-and-rebuild stage starts within hours after the initial injury, it can actually take several months for the body to be fully healed. During the repair-and-rebuild process, skin cells start migrating across the wound, while collagen and new blood vessels are being laid down underneath, weaving your new tissue.

Stage 4: Maturation. Connective tissue and skin can be remodeled in three to four months, while bone takes longer—up to two years for the minerals to be laid down in its matrix.

MANAGING THE ACID-ALKALINE BALANCE

Being nutritionally fit for healing will not only help you heal faster, but will decrease the pain. The best tool you have for healing is the way you choose to eat. For instance, a diet high in sugar is acidic, whereas incorporating alkalinizing foods, such as lemons, limes and dark leafy greens, are loaded with vitamins, minerals, and antioxidants that combat the acidity.

The book, *Conscious Eating*, a wonderful publication written by Gabriel Cousens, MD, contains detailed information about the effect of food on health. Dr. Cousens explains clearly why it is important to maintain a healthy acid-alkaline balance so the enzymes and cells in the body can function optimally. The human body maintains a constant blood pH of 7.4, which is considered to be a neutral balance of acidity to alkaline.

There are two ways to test pH: through urine or saliva. In urine samples, normal pH should be between 6.8 and 7.5; in saliva, the ideal pH level should be 7.4. While there is a large range of acceptable pH in medical literature, usually between 6.2 and 7.2, optimum pH lies between 7 and 7.4. If oral pH drops below 5.5, then teeth begin to demineralize, resulting in cavities and potential teeth fractures.

The best way to check pH at home is by using litmus strips, which can be purchased online or at any pharmacy or natural foods store. The most accurate results will appear if urine or saliva is tested in the morning before any food is consumed. Monitoring pH diligently will inform you of your body's acid-alkaline balance, which may lean towards acidity if you are recovering from illness or disease, or if you are under a lot of stress. An acidic pH level often results in symptoms such as inflammation, anxiety, aggressiveness, fatigue, and muscle spasms.

If your acid-alkaline balance is off, the remedy is to change your diet. Here are a few tips to alkalinize your body so that optimum healing can occur:

- Eat more food in the alkaline zone (see chart)

- Eat more sprouted foods

- Add lemon or lime juice to your diet

- Drink green juice and wheatgrass juice

- Take plant enzymes to enhance digestion

- Decrease intake of sugar, alcohol, and processed foods

- Decrease intake of animal protein

- Decrease intake of unhealthy fats

- Decrease dairy intake

Although rare, it is possible for blood to have a tendency to become alkaline. Too much alkaline can cause symptoms such as headaches, depression, mood swings, aggression, and bad breath. If your tested urinary or salivary pH is above 7.2, then you may also use food to repair the balance. Here are a few quick remedies:

- Drink raw, organic apple cider vinegar

- Increase protein intake

- Increase fat intake

- Eat fermented foods, such as sauerkraut

- Eat more acid-forming foods (see chart)

NEUTRAL & ACID
FORMING FOODS

NEUTRAL······SLIGHTLY ACID········MOD ACID········EXTREMELY ACID FORMING

NEUTRAL	SLIGHTLY ACID		MOD ACID		EXTREMELY ACID FORMING		
• Butter, fresh unsalted	• Blueberries	• Barley malt syrup	• Bananas, green & tasty	• Cigarette tobacco, roll your own	• Beer	• Beef	• Artificial sweeteners
• Cream, fresh & raw	• Brazil nuts	• Barley	• Buckwheat	• Cream of wheat, unrefined	• Brown sugar	• Carbonated soft drinks & fizzy drinks	
• Margarine	• Butter, salted	• Bran	• Cheeses, sharp		• Chicken		
• Milk, raw cow's	• Cheeses, mild & crumbly	• Cashews	• Corn & rice breads	• Fish	• Deer	• Cigarettes, tailor-made	
• Oils (except olive)	• Crackers, unrefined rye	• Cereals, unrefined with honey fruit or maple syrup	• Egg, whole (cooked hard)	• Fruit juices with sugar	• Chocolate	• Drugs	
• Whey, cow's	• Dried beans mung, adzuki, pinto, kidney, garbanzo	• Cornmeal	• Ketchup	• Maple syrup, processed	• Coffee	• Flour, white wheat	
• Yoghurt, plain		• Cranberries	• Mayonaise	• Molasses, sulphured	• Custard with white sugar	• Goat	
	• Dry coconut	• Fructose	• Oats	• Pickles, commercial	• Jellies	• Lamb	
	• Egg whites	• Honey, pasteurized	• Pasta, whole grains & honey	• Breads (refined) of corn, oats, rice & rye	• Jams	• Pastries & cakes from white flour	
	• Goat's milk, homogenised	• Lentils	• Pastry, wholegrain		• Liquor	• Pork	
	• Olives, pickled	• Macadamias	• Peanuts	• Cereals (refined) eg weetbix, corn flakes	• Pasta, white	• Sugar, white	
	• Pecans	• Maple syrup, unprocessed	• Popcorn, with salt & butter		• Rabbit		
	• Plums	• Milk, homogenized, & most processed dairy products	• Rice, basmati	• Shellfish	• Semolina		
	• Prunes		• Rice, brown	• Wheatgerm	• Table salt, refined & iodised		
	• Spelt	• Molasses, unsulph -ered organic	• Soy sauce, commercial	• Whole Wheat foods	• Tea, black		
		• Nutmeg	• Tapioca	• Wine	• Turkey		
		• Mustard	• Wheatbread, sprouted organic	• Yoghurt, sweetened	• Wheat bread		
		• Pistachios			• White rice		
		• Popcorn & butter, plain			• White vinegar, processed		
		• Rice or wheat crackers, unrefined					
		• Rye, grain					
		• Ryebread, organic sprouted					
		• Seeds, pumpkins & sunflower					
		• Walnuts					

ALKALINE
FORMING FOODS

MOST ALKALINE FORMING·············MODERATE····················SLIGHTLY···········

MOST ALKALINE FORMING			MODERATE			SLIGHTLY	
• Lemons	• Agar Agar	• Asparagus	• Apples, sweet	• Apples, sour	• Almonds	• Amaranth	
• Watermelon	• Cantaloupe	• Endive	• Apricots	• Bamboo shoots	• Artichokes, Jerusalem	• Artichoke, globe	
	• Cayenne	• Kiwifruit	• Alfalfa sprouts	• Beans, fresh green	• Barley-Malt, sweetner - Bronner	• Chestnuts, dry roasted	
	• Dried dates & figs	• Fruit juices	• Arrowroot flour	• Beets		• Egg yolks, soft cooked	
	• Kelp, Karengo	• Grapes, sweet	• Avocados	• Bell pepper	• Brown Rice Syrup	• Essene bread	
	• Kudzu root	• Passionfruit	• Bananas, ripe	• Broccoli	• Brussel Sprouts	• Goat's milk & whey, raw	
	• Limes	• Pears, sweet	• Berries	• Cabbage; Cauli	• Cherries	• Horseradish	
	• Mango	• Pineapple	• Carrots	• Carob	• Coconut, fresh	• Mayonaise, home-made	
	• Melons	• Raisins	• Celery	• Daikon	• Cucumbers	• Millet	
	• Papaya	• Umeboshi plum	• Currants	• Ginger, fresh	• Egg plant	• Olive oil	
	• Parsley	• Vegetable juices	• Dates & Figs, fresh	• Grapes, sour	• Honey, raw	• Quinoa	
	• Seedless grapes; sweet		• Garlic	• Kale	• Leeks	• Rhubarb	
	• Watercress		• Gooseberry	• Kohlrabi	• Miso	• Sesame seeds, whole	
	• Seaweeds		• Grapes, less sweet	• Lettuce, pale green	• Mushrooms	• Soy beans, dry	
			• Grapefruit	• Oranges	• Okra	• Soy cheese	
			• Guavas	• Parsnip	• Olives ripe	• Soy milk	
			• Herbs, leafy green	• Peaches, less sweet	• Onions	• Sprouted grains	
			• Lettuce, leafy green	• Peas, less sweet	• Pickles, home made	• Tempeh	
			• Nectarine	• Potatoes & skin	• Radish	• Tofu	
			• Peaches, sweet	• Pumpkin, less sweet	• Sea salt	• Tomatoes, less sweet	
			• Pears, less sweet	• Rasberry	• Spices	• Yeast, nutritional flakes	
			• Peas, fresh, sweet	• Sapote	• Taro		
			• Persimmon	• Strawberry	• Tomatoes, sweet		
			• Pumpkin, sweet	• Squash	• Vinegar, sweet brown rice		
			• Sea salt, vegetable	• Sweet corn, fresh	• Water Chestnuts		
			• Spinach	• Tamari			
				• Turnip			
				• Vinegar,			

When facing surgery, the body has a tendency to become relatively acidic, and needs more alkaline-forming foods to regain balance. Alkaline-forming foods, such as lemon and lime, can be very acidic, an especially important point when it comes to oral surgery as the wound will come into direct contact with any ingested foods. Acidic foods that come into contact with any intraoral wound can sensitize the nerve endings and cause persistent pain. Anyone with intraoral ulcers should opt for more neutral foods, such as:

- Coconut juice

- Aloe vera

- Avocado

- Cucumber

- Celery

- Apple

- Grapes

- Melons

Other foods to avoid for efficient healing of intraoral ulcers include:

- Citrus fruits

- Tomatoes

- Pineapple

Fat is another extremely necessary nutrient that can help with the acid-alkaline balance. Recent studies have shown that having fat in the diet promotes healing and provides a fuel source to the mito-chondria, or powerhouses, of cells. Additionally, both bone marrow and olive oil can greatly contribute to the alkalization of the body.

SUGAR EFFECTS

As I mentioned in the introduction, chronic inflammation is a global epidemic. It is a common malady that can lead to cardiovascular disease, obesity, diabetes, high cholesterol, rheumatoid arthritis, periodontitis, and many other diseases and conditions. However, a healthy diet, which includes nearly eliminating sugar consumption, can prevent chronic inflammation.

Most individuals do not realize how many foods today are rife with sugar; some statistics say that up to 20 percent of ingested calories come from processed sugars. High levels of sugar in the body create the perfect habitat and incubator for viruses, yeasts, and even cancer cells.

Sugar also causes havoc in the mouth by increasing the rate of cavities or caries. This is the most common and preventable oral disease. The mouth paints a picture of what is happening to the rest of the body, so if the teeth are diseased, so, too, is the inside of the body.

Research has shown that dental cavities form not only as a direct result of sugar touching the tooth, but because of the interruption of nourishing fluids that flow to the tooth. This occurs when there is a disturbance in the brain caused by high sugar intake.

High sugar intake creates an increase in oxidative stress in the brain, which makes the tooth vulnerable to oral bacteria. To the tooth, eating sugar is a bit like a river that finally stops flowing: before long, the riverbed will begin to appear muddy and there will be an overgrowth of organisms. On the tooth, bacteria consume the sugar and produce an acid byproduct, which ultimately erodes the tooth surface and causes cavities. During this time, saliva becomes critical to neutralizing the acid produced by the bacteria. Eating foods rich in vitamin K2, such as natto or fermented cheeses, can remineralize damaged teeth by releasing more calcium and inorganic phosphates in saliva.

MAINTAINING BLOOD SUGAR AND OPTIMUM HEALTH

Mark Hyman, MD, author of *The Blood Sugar Solution*, explains the importance of maintaining a constant blood sugar level in order to achieve optimum health.

A more optimal level of health can be reached by consuming strictly low-glycemic foods; foods are ranked on the Glycemic Index (GI) by how they affect blood sugar levels. Foods that have a high glycemic index enter the body and cause a spike in blood sugar levels, which can lead to chronic inflammation, degenerative diseases, and poor wound healing.

A high-glycemic index can be found in white flour, sugar, potatoes, bread, and breakfast cereals. Even some fruits contain a high-glycemic index and should be eaten only in moderation. Sweetened beverages such as fruit juices should be avoided altogether, as these provide too much sugar all at once. The GI of foods should be included on labels, so one can make better choices, especially when it comes to controlling type 2 diabetes. It is difficult to calculate the GI from the food label. As a general rule, look at the carbohydrate content to be as low as possible and the fiber content to be higher.

IN PLACE OF SUGAR

While sugary and processed foods can spike blood sugar levels, removing them entirely from the diet can be a challenge. In place of sugar, there are a number of sugar substitutes that can be used as healthy alternatives and that do not always possess a high GI. Here are a few:

Xylitol is one of these wonderful replacements. Xylitol is a natural extract from birch tree cellulose, also found in other fruits and vegetables, which has been used as a natural sweetener throughout history. For instance, during World War II in Finland, to compensate for a sugar shortage, the Finnish started substituting with xylitol from the birch trees scattered throughout the country. As an unintended result, there was a significant decrease in cavities nationwide. Studies have shown that xylitol promotes the growth of healthy bacteria, and can even reduce child ear infections by up to 30 percent. Xylitol can be found today as a white granular powder, or in the form of candy and chewing gum, and is a great option for children and adults who wish to regulate the balance between internal bacteria. Xylitol is best consumed in small quantities, as larger amounts may cause gas in some people.

Erythrol is another sugar substitute from the same family as xylitol. Like xylitol, erythrol is free of calories and does not raise the blood sugar level when consumed. While it has similar properties to xylitol, it is more difficult to find commercially and may only be available in specialty stores—although it is becoming a popular sweetener in certain beverages that are readily available on the market. Unlike xylitol, erythrol is produced via fermentation, and will not cause the unfortunate GI-based side effects that are common in some people who ingest xylitol.

Honey, a practical superfood, remains as one of the healthiest alternatives to sugar. Organic, raw, unfiltered honey is rich in antioxidants, minerals, and enzymes that possess tremendous anti-inflammatory and healing properties. Consuming large amounts of honey raises blood sugar levels, so diabetics should limit the intake. Honey is a great treatment for sore throats and other throat-related maladies. Wild honey has also been used to treat other diseases such as irritable bowel syndrome, stomach ulcers, and other infections. Even the topical use of honey has been around since Egyptian times, being used to heal wounds such as burns, cuts, abscesses, surgical incisions, diabetic ulcers, and skin infections. When selecting honey, search for wild, raw honey, or raw organic honey that has been stored in a translucent glass container. Consume in small quantities, such as one or two teaspoons a day due to its high glycemic index.

Manuka honey, a varietal from New Zealand, retains antifungal, antiviral, and even antibiotic properties, and is a great remedy for oral ulcers. A teaspoon of Manuka honey applied to an oral ulcer is a great home remedy.

Stevia is one of the most widely available sugar substitutes. Stevia is a calorie-free extract from a South African herb that is safe for diabetics or individuals with blood sugar problems. While it is an excellent alternative, it is two hundred times sweeter than sugar, and contains an aftertaste that may be displeasing to some. Stevia can be found in the form of drops, powder, and even crushed leaves. In recent studies, stevia has been found to have antibacterial properties.

Monk fruit or sweetfruit drops are another fantastic sugar substitute. It comes from the Chinese tonic herb, Luo Han Guo. The drops not only sweeten food, but also support the immune system, due to their high levels of saponin, a foamy plant chemical. Sweetfruit drops are three hundred times sweeter than refined sugar, yet contain only 5 percent of the calories and have no known negative side effects. These can be found at a natural food store as a tincture or powder.

Agave is another substitute for sugar, yet there has been much controversy surrounding this cactus-based sweetener. It can be used as a way to abandon sugar but has a high-fructose content and should only be used sparingly, as it is hard on the liver. Agave does come in a syrupy form and is a delicious addition to any foods needing an extra dose of sweetener.

Trehalose is another natural sugar substitute that is found in mushrooms, drought-resistant plants, bacteria, insects, and also animal meat. Recent studies have shown that this sweetener can prevent bone loss, and can also help cells retain water in periods of dehydration. Trehalose is available commercially and has even appeared in a variety of different sports drinks.

Artificial sweeteners have been used for years as a replacement for regular sugar and are still being widely used. Unfortunately, these artificial alternatives often contain aspartame, a substance that has been shown to cause side effects such as headaches, blurry vision, and even obesity. Sucralose is toxic to the liver and can cause liver enlargement, as well as lymphatic system blockage. Artificial sweeteners should be avoided by anyone wishing to keep a healthy lifestyle.

As a former sugar addict, I know just how hard it is to start making changes and getting rid of those high sugary foods. After all, sugar is a drug and your brain is on it. I suggest you gradually start the switch away from sugary foods so you don't go through an uncomfortable withdrawal that could include low energy, headaches, and moodiness. Try replacing regular sugar with one of the substitutes above and notice you will start to feel better.

Since sugary and processed foods alter the taste buds, it can be difficult to make the switch to fresh, natural foods. But there is a solution—spices.

DON'T FORGET YOUR SPICES!

Fresh foods are good for you and taste wonderful, but their health benefits can be enhanced even further by the simple inclusion of a few spices.

Researchers all over the world have been analyzing spices for decades, and have only begun to understand the true healing properties of these delicious, dried delicacies. Turmeric, cloves, and coriander have been employed for ages, as they contain anti-inflammatory phytonutrients and oils that are not present in other foods. Phytonutrients, or phytochemicals, are compounds produced by plants to help them thrive or ward off predators and pathogens. They have been shown to help reduce the risk of chronic disease and inflammation. Some researchers estimate that there are approximately four thousand phytonutrients, but only a small number have been studied in detail. Here are some of the more common anti-inflammatory spices.

Turmeric, commonly found in curry, is an extremely powerful spice. It can be identified by its rich, yellow color, and contains an active ingredient known as curcumin, a substance proven to have anti-inflammatory and antioxidizing capabilities. Studies have shown that this spice can decrease, and even eliminate, the symptoms of chronic inflammation. Turmeric, added to the diet, can aid against productions of free radicals. Turmeric supplementation may also help protect the brain and the spinal cord against free radical damage, and may shield the blood vessels—including the small blood vessels in the back of the eye—from oxidative damage. Curcumin has been studied extensively and has been shown to provide anti-cancer benefits by slowing down the growth of cancerous cells. Curcumin protects against radiation, inflammation, and neurodegeneration, such as in Alzheimer's.

Cloves also deserve a notable mention in the battle against inflammation. The eugenol in cloves has a long history of use in dentistry as an analgesic agent. Cloves can be kept in the kitchen and, used accordingly, for pain relief. Clove oil can be found over the counter and it can be applied straight to the area to relieve oral pain. Only a small amount is necessary.

Coriander, the seeds of cilantro, contains fiber, calcium, selenium, iron, magnesium, and manganese. Coriander essential oil has been shown to inhibit the growth of Staph aureus, E. coli, and other bacteria. I will discuss essential oils and their benefits in chapter 5.

Cumin, commonly found in Indian food, has strong immune-boosting abilities.

Ground pepper, a widely used spice in cuisines throughout the world, can be beneficial in protecting brain cells. It's extract, bioperine, is often used in supplements as an anti-inflammatory agent.

Fenugreek is less commonly known, but it is found in many Asian dishes, and has been shown to improve or relieve symptoms of arthritis.

Allspice is shown to have 25 different phenols that can help fight oxidative stress that results in cellular damage. Some studies have shown that it can even help with menopause, osteoporosis, and with the overall lowering of blood pressure.

There are many other spices that can also be used as healthy supplements in the human body.

HERB	FORM OF USE	NUTRIENTS	THERAPEUTIC EFFECT
Acerola berry	Fruit, powder, capsule	Rich in **vitamin C**, also A, Bs, calcium, iron, magnesium	Antioxidant, antifungal, great for skin and soft tissue healing
Alfa-alfa	Sprouts	phytonutrients (lutein, zeaxanthin, genistein etc.), calcium, magnesium, copper, iron, zinc, vitamin A, Bs, C, D, E, and K.	Alkalinizes, anti-inflammatory, digestion, balances blood sugar and cholesterol, bone density
Aloe	Pulp from leaves, liquid, gel, capsule	Phytonutrients (saponins, beta-caroteen, lignins etc.), amino acids, calcium, folate, iron, magnesium, zinc, vitamin A, Bs, C, E	Antibacterial, antiviral, anti-inflammatory, laxative, heals mouth and stomach ulcers, digestion
Anise	Seeds, oil, flavoring	Phytonutrients, calcium, iron, magnesium, manganese, phosphorous, potassium, zinc, vitamin A, Bs, C, E	Digestion, promotes breast milk production, good for respiratory infections
Annatto	Whole plant, seeds, food coloring	Phytonutrients (beta caroteen, salicylic acid, tannins etc.), amino acids, calcium, iron, phosphorous, vitamin C	Antioxidant, antibacterial, anti-inflammatory, digestion, skin care, expectorant

Ashwagandha (indian ginseng, winter cherry)	Roots, capsules, powder, tea	Phytonutrients, amino acids, choline	Anti-inflammatory, immune support, adaptogen, stress support, improves physical endurance and sexual function
Astragalus	Roots, tea, powder, capsules	Phytonutrients (betaine etc.), calcium, copper, iron, magnesium, manganese, potassium, zinc, essential fatty acids, choline	Immune support, adaptogen, stress support, digestion, **healing,** energy,
Bilberry (european blueberry	Whole plant, tea, tincture, dietary supplement	Phytonutrients (anthocyanins, beta carotene, ferulic acid, lutein, quercetin), calcium, magnesium, manganese, phosphorous, potassium, selenium, silicon, sulphur, zinc, vitamin C	Antioxidant, anti-inflammatory, improves circulation by adding flexibility to blood vessels, connective tissue, collagen support, anti-carcinogenic, eye health
Birch	Leaves, tea, ground bark, sap (drink), syrup	Phytonutrients (betulin, quercetin, methyl salicylate, etc.)	Anti-inflammatory, diuretic, anti-carcinogenic, **pain reliever, especially joint pain**
Black cohosh	Roots as a dietary supplement, capsules	Phytonutrients (beta carotene, salicylic acid, tannin etc.), calcium, chromium, iron, magnesium, manganese, phosphorous, potassium, selenium, zinc, silicon	Decreases symptoms of menopause, lowers blood pressure, mucus, cholesterol, improves osteoporosis

Black walnut	Bark, leaves, tea,	Beta carotene, tannins, calcium, iron, manganese, magnesium, phosphorous, potassium, selemium, zinc, vitamin B6, C, E, silicon	Antifungal, antiviral, anti-carcinogenic, heals mouth ulcers,
Borage	Leaves, oil from seeds, capsules	Phytonutrients (beta-carotene, rosmarinic acid, tannin), calcium, choline, EFAs, iron, magnesium, zinc, vitamin C	Cardiovascular function, healthy skin, adrenal tonic
Boswellia (indian frankincense)	Resin as powder, capsules	Phytonutrients (borneol, geraniol, linomene)	Anti-inflammatory, anti-fungal, antibacterial, topical pain relief, blood vessels repair
Burdock	Roots, seeds, capsules, tea	Phytonutrients (acetic acid, arctiin, beta-carotene, inulin, etc.), amino acids, calcium, phosphorous, potassium, selenium, zinc, vitamin C	Antioxidant, anti-carcinogenic, antibacterial, antifungal, detoxifying.
Calendula (marigold)	Flowers, lotion, tincture	Phytonutrients (alpha-amyrin, lutein, quercetin, rutin etc.), calcium, CoQ10, vitamin C, E	Anti-inflammatory, heals skin scrapes, burns, rashes, calming for toothaches and nerve pain
Catnip	Leaves, tea, capsules, tincture	Phytonutrients (camphor, thymol etc.), calcium, iron, chromium, magnesium, manganese, phosphorous, potassium, selenium, zinc	Anti-inflammatory, anti-anxiety, sleep aid, treats headaches

Cat's claw	Bark, leaves, tea, capsules	Phytonutrients (allopteropodine, ursolic acid etc.), enzymes that convert saturated fat to unsaturated fat	Antioxidant, anti-inflammatory, stimulates immune system, detoxifies the intestines
Cayenne (hot pepper, red pepper)	Seeds and fruit, spice, lotion, tincture	Phytonutrients (alpha and beta carotene, capsaicin, lutein, zeaxanthin etc.), calcium, EFA, folate, magnesium, zinc, vitamin C, E, Bs	Improves circulation, digestion, stops bleeding, helps with pain
Celery	Whole plant and seeds	Phytonutrients (eugenol, ferulic acid, limonene, ruin etc.), boron, choline, amino acids, folate, inositol, iron, magnesium, manganese, phosphorous, potassium, selenium, sulfur, zinc, vitamin A, Bs, C, E, K	Reduces blood pressure, muscle spasms, antioxidant
Chamomile	Flowers, tea, tincture, mouthwash	Phytonutrients (alpha-bisabolol, quercetin, rutin, tannin, etc.), choline, vitamin C	Anti-inflammatory, calming, pain reduction, sleep aid, reduces mouth/gum infections
Cinnamon	Bark, plant, spice, tea	Phytonutrients (alpha-pinene, linalool, mucilage, etc.), calcium, copper, iodine, iron, manganese, phosphorous, potassium, zinc, vitamin A, Bs, C.	Anti-inflammatory, anti-fungal, digestion, controls blood sugar.

Clove	Flower buds, seeds, oil, spice, tincture	Phytonutrients (beta-carotene, beta-pinene, eugenol, mucilage, tannin etc.), calcium, iron, magnesium, manganese, potassium, zinc, vitamin A, Bs, C	Oral antiseptic, anti-parasitic
Comfrey	Whole plant extract, lotion, tincture, oil	Phytonutrients (allantoin, rosmarinic acid etc.), calcium, iron, magnesium, manganese, phosphorous, potassium, selenium, zinc, vitamin Bs and C	Speeds **wound healing,** bedsores, bites, bruises, rashes. External use only.
Corn silk	Tea	Phytonutrients (betaine, caffeic acid, carotene, glycol acid, thymol, etc.), calcium, iron, magnesium, potassium, phosphorour, vitamin C	Diuretic, decreases edema
Cranberry	Fruit, powder, capsules	Phytonutrients (alpha-terpineol, carotene, eugenol, ferulic acid, malic acid, quercetin etc.), calcium, magnesium, manganese, iron, folate, potassium, selenium, sulfur, zinc, vitamin A, Bs, C, E	Antioxidant, anti-carcinogenic, helpful for urinary infections, improves memory
Dandelion	Whole plant, powder, capsules, tincture	Phytonutrients (carotenes, caffeic acid, saponin etc.), calcium, iron, magnesium, manganese, potassium, phosphorous, selenium, zinc, vitamin Bs, C	Detoxifier, anti-inflammatory, increases bile production, helps with stomach problems

Echinacea	Whole plant, tea, capsules, tincture	Phytonutrients (alpha-pinene, carotene, betaine, quercetin, rutin etc.), calcium, magnesium, manganese, potassium, Phosphorous, selenium, zinc, vitamin C	Anti-inflammatory, antibacterial, antiviral, stimulates immune system
Elderberry (elder)	Fruit, flowers, capsules, syrup, tincture, preserves, liquor	Phytonutrients (alpha-amyrin, astragal, betulin, etc.), EFAs, vitamin A, Bs, C	Anti-inflammatory, stimulates immune system, helps treat respiratory infections, skin irritations
Fennel	Whole plant and seeds, spice	Phytonutrients 9 alpha-pinene, carotene, camphor, quercetin etc.), calcium, magnesium, iron, manganese, phosphorous, potassium, selenium, vitamin B, C, E, amino acids, EFAs	Digestion and abdominal pain reliever, GI distress.
Fenugreek	Seeds, oil, spice	Phytonutrients (beta-carotene, coumarin, quercetin, rutin, saponin etc.), amino acids, calcium, magnesium, iron, manganese, phosphorous, potassium, selenium, zinc, vitamin C	Laxative, fever reducer, anti-inflammatory for eyes and lungs
Flax	Seeds, oil, ground supplement	Phytonutrients (apigenin, beta-carotene, lecithin, etc.), amino acids, EFAs, iron, magnesium, manganese, phosphorous, potassium, sulphur, vanadium, zinc, vitamin Bs, E	Strengthens collagen for bones, nails, teeth, skin, anti-inflammatory

Garlic	Bulb, capsules, oil	Phytonutrients (allicin, carotene, ferulic acid, quercetin, rutin etc), calcium, folate, iron, magnesium, manganese, potassium, selenium, zinc, vitamin Bs, C	Antibacterial, antiparasitic, stimulates immune system, lowers blood pressure, stomach ulcers (kills H. Pylori)
Ginger	Roots, powder, spice, capsules, tea, candy	Phytonutrients (alpha-pinene, camphor, capsaicin, curcumin, lecithin, etc.), amino acids, calcium, EFAs, iron, manganese, selenium, zinc, vitamin A, C, E	Anti-inflammatory, antispasmodic, antioxidant, antimicrobial, aids in stomach pain, nausea, vomiting
Gingko	Leaves, seeds, powder, tea, capsules, tincture	Phytonutrients (amoentoflavones, quercetin, tannins, etc.), calcium, magnesium, iron, manganese, phosphorous, potassium, zinc, vitamin A, Bs, C	Improves circulation and tissue oxygenation. Antioxidant. Beneficial for tinnitus.
Ginseng	Roots, tea, powder, capsules	Phytonutrients (beta-sitosterol, escin, saponin etc.), calcium, choline, folate, iron, magnesium, manganese, silicone, zinc, vitamin Bs and C	Supports immune system, circulation, stamina, protects against radiation
Goldenseal	Roots, capsules, tea, tincture	Phytonutrients (berberine, carrotene, etc.), calcium, iron, magnesium, phosphorous, potassium, selenium, zinc, vitamin C	Anti-inflammatory, antimicrobial, supports immune system

Gotu kola	Nuts, roots, oil, capsules	Phytonutrients (carotene, camphor, saponin etc.), calcium, iron, magnesium, selenium, zinc	Speeds **wound healing,** decreases fatigue, edema
Green tea	Leaves, powder, spice, capsules	Phytonutrients (apigenin, astragalin, carotene, eugenol, lutein, myristic acid, quercetin, salycilic acid, thymol, zeaxanthin), calcium, iron, magnesium, manganese, potassium, zinc, vitamin C, Bs.	Antioxidant, anti-carcinogenic, lowers cholesterol, stimulates immune system, fights cavities
Guarana	Seeds, powder, beverages, energy drinks, tea, capsules	Phytonutrients (adenine, caffeine, tannins etc.)	Tonic, stamina, endurance
Hops	Flowers and leaves, tea, capsule	Phytonutrients (alpha-pinene, carotene, catechin, eugenol etc.), calcium, magnesium, zinc, vitamin C	Antibacterial, antifungal, sleep aid, helps relieve pain, toothache
Horse chestnut	Leaves, seeds, bark, oil, tincture, lotion	Phytonutrients (allantoin, esculin, fraxin, quercetin, rutin etc.)	Topical use reduces pain, swelling, bruising
Irish moss	Whole plant, thickener in cooking	Phytonutrients (beta-carotene), calcium, iron, magnesium, manganese, selenium, zinc, vitamin Bs and C	Expectorant, emolient for dry skin and hair

Juniper	Fruit, tincture, gin	Phytonutrients (alpha-pinene, botulin, camphor, catechin, monthol, tannins etc.), calcium, iron, magnesium, manganese, phosphorous, potassium, selenium, zinc, vitamin Bs and C	Anti-inflammatory, diuretic, regulates blood sugar level
Kava kava	Roots, powder, capsules, tea	Phytonutrients (cinnamic acid, kavalolactones, etc.)	Relaxation, GI calm, analgesic
Kudzu	Leaves, roots, food starch	Phytonutrients (daidzein, genistein, quercetin etc.), calcium, iron, magnesium, phosphorous, potassium, vitamin B2	Lowers BP and tinnitus, relieves headaches
Lavender	Flowers, tea, spice, tincture, oil	Phytonutrients (alpha-pinene, camphor, tannin etc.)	Calming, relieves headaches, aids with skin problems.
Lemongrass	Stems, spice, tea, tincture, capsules, oil	Phytonutrients (alpha-pinene, limonene, linalool, etc.), calcium, iron, magnesium, manganese, phosphorous, potassium, selenium, zinc	Analgesic, antimicrobial, antiseptic, antifungal, digestive aid, tonic
Licorice	Roots, capsules, tea, tincture	Phytonutrients (apigenin, carotene, betaine, camphor, eugenol, quercetin etc.), calcium, choline, iron, magnesium, manganese, phosphorous, potassium, selenium, zinc, vitamin Bs and C	Anti-inflammatory, antiviral, antiparasitic and antibacterial, has estrogen/ progesterone like effect, decreases dental plaque, decreases pain.

Maca	Roots, powder, tea, capsules	Phytonutrients (beta-sitosterol, saponin, tannins etc.), calcium, iron, magnesium, phosphorous, zinc, vitamin B12, C, E	Increases energy and fertility
Milk thistle	Fruit, leaves, seeds, capsules, tincture	Phytonutrients (apigenin, carotene, fumaric acid, quercetin, silymarin etc.), calcium, iron, magnesium, manganese, phosphorous, potassium, selenium, zinc	Liver detoxification and regeneration
Mustard	Seeds, condiment, topical oil	Phytonutrients (allyl isothiocyanate, Ferulic acid, etc.)	Digestive aid, topical anti-inflammatory for joints and trauma
Myrrh	Resin, tincture	Phytonutrients (acetic acid, eugenol, etc.)	Antiseptic, antiviral, antibacterial, treatment of bad breath, cold sores and periodontal disease
Nettle	Whole plant, cooking, tea, capsules	Phytonutrients (acetic acid, carotene, betaine, lycopene etc.), calcium, copper, iron, magnesium, manganese, phosphorous, potassium, selenium, Sulphur, zinc, vitamin Bs, C	Pain relief, tonic, anti-inflammatory
Olive leaf	Leaves, capsules, tincture	Phytonutrients (apigenin, mannitol, quercetin, rutin, tannins etc.), calcium	Antibacterial, antiviral, anti-fungal, anti-parasitic, antioxidant

Oregano - wild	Stems, spice, tincture	Phytonutrients (alpha-pinene, apigenin, carotene, catechol, eugenol, quercetin, thymol, vitexin, etc.), calcium, iron, magnesium, phosphorous, potassium, zinc, vitamin A, Bs, C	Anti-inflammatory, antibacterial, antiparasitic, antifungal, antiviral, supports the immune system.
Papaya	Fruit, leaves, seeds, capsules, seeds as a spice	Phytonutrients (benzaldehyge, carotene, lycopene, papain, zeaxanthin), calcium, iron, magnesium, manganese, phosphorous, potassium, zinc	Antiinflammatory, aids in digestion
Parsley	Whole plant	Phytonutrients (alpha-pinene, carotene, lutein, myristic acid, etc.), calcium, iron, magnesium, manganese, phosphorous, potassium, selenium, zinc, vitamin A, Bs, C, E	Antitumorigenic, antiinflammatory, aids in bad breath
Passionflower	Whole plant	Phytonutrients (apigenin, flavonoids, quercetin, rutin, etc.), calcium, amino acids	Relieves anxiety and stress
Pau d'arco	Bark, tea	Phytonutrients (beta-carotene, lapachol, etc.)	Antibacterial, antifungal, treatment of oral candidiasis
Pepper			
Peppermint	Leaves, flowers, oil, tea, flavoring	Phytonutrients (acetic acid, carotene, alpha-pinene, eugenol, etc.)	Pain relief,anti- nausea

Primrose	Seeds, oil, capsules	Phytonutrients (beta-sitosterol, lignin, quercetin etc.), calcium, EFAs, iron, magnesium, manganese, phosphorous, potassium, zinc, vitamin E	Treatment of eczema and nerve pain
Red raspberries	Leaves and roots	Phytonutrients (carotene, ferulic acid, lutein, tannin etc.), calcium, iron, magnesium, manganese phosphorous, potassium, selenium, silicon, zinc, vitamin Bs, C, E	Strengthens teeth, bone, nails, skin, anti-nausea, reduces intestinal cramps
Rhubarb	Roots and stalks	Phytonutrients (acetic acid, carotene, lutein, rutin, etc.), calcium, iron, magnesium, manganese, phosphorous, potassium, selenium, sulphur	Anti-inflammatory, anti-parasitic, laxative
Rose hips	Fruit, preserves, tea, tincture, capsules	Phytonutrients (carotene, catechin, flavonoids, lycopene, zeaxanthin etc.), calcium, iron, magnesium, manganese, phosphorous, potassium, selenium, zinc, vitamin Bs, C, E	Antioxidant, anti-diarrhea,

Rosemary	Leaves, spice, oil, tincture	Phytonutrients (alpha-pinene, apigenin, carotene, camphor, geraniol, salicylates, thymol, etc.), calcium, iron, magnesium, manganese, phosphorous, potassium, zinc, vitamin Bs, C	Anti-inflammatory, antibacterial, anti-fungal, antioxidant, antiseptic mouthwash, anticarcinogenic
Sage	Leaves, spice, oil, tea	Phytonutrients (alpha-amyrin, carotene, betulin, camphor, tannins, saponin, etc.), boron, calcium, iron, magnesium, manganese, phosphorous, potassium, selenium, zinc, vitamin Bs, C	Anti-inflammatory, especially oral inflammation
Sangre de grado (dragon's blood)	Bark, resin, tincture, tea	Phytonutrients (Alpha-pinene, betaine, eugenol, tannins, etc.)	Antioxidant, anti-inflammatory, antibacterial, antiviral, anti fungal. **Aids in wound healing and mouth ulcers,** stops bleeding.
Skullcap	Leaves, capsules, tincture	Phytonutrients (carotene, lignin, tannins), calcium, iron, magnesium, manganese, phosphorous, potassium, selenium, zinc, vitamin Bs, C	Promotes sleep, relieves pain, cramps, spasms, anxiety
Thyme	Leaves, flowers, spice, oil, tea infusion	Phytonutrients (alpha-pinene, apigenin, carotene, camphor, geraniol, salicylates, thymol, etc.), Ca, Fe, Mg, Mn, P, K, Zn, Vit Bs and C.	Antibacterial, anti fungal, good for respiratory infections

Turmeric	Root, tea, powder, capsules, seasoning	Phytonutrients (alpha-pinene, carotene, curcumin, eugenol, turmerone, etc.), calcium, iron, manganese, phosphorous, potassium, zinc, vitamin Bs, C	Anti-inflammatory, blood thinner, antibiotic, anticancer
Valerian	Root, tea, tincture, capsules	Phytonutrients (azulene, carotene, valeric acid, etc.), calcium, iron, magnesium, zinc, phosphorous, potassium, selenium, vitamin Bs, C, choline, EFAs,	Sedative, improves circulation
White oak	Bark, tea, tincture, capsules	Phytonutrients (carotene, catechin, quercetin, tannins etc.), calcium, iron, magnesium, manganese, phosphorous, potassium, selenium, zinc, vitamin Bs, C	Anti-inflammatory, antiseptic, topical and oral applications, anti-diarrhea
White willow	Bark, tea, tincture, capsules	Phytonutrients (apigenin, carotene, catechin, lignin, salicin, salicylic acid etc.), calcium, iron, magnesium, manganese, phosphorous, potassium, selenium, zinc, vitamin Bs, C	Reduces pain and fever, aspirin like effect
Wintergreen	Whole plant, oil for flavoring	Phytonutrients (caffeic acid, ferulic acid, gallic acid, methyl salicylate)	Anti-inflammatory, relieves pain, headaches, toothache, aspirin like effects
Witch hazel	Bark, leaves, tincture, powder	Phytonutrients (beto-ionone, gallic acid, phenol, quercetin etc.)	Anti-inflammatory, Healing to oral wounds.

Wormwood	Leaves, tincture, tea, spice	Phytonutrients (carotene, rutin, salicylic acid, etc.), vitamin C	Anti-parasitic, antifungal, antimicrobial, anti-carcinogenic, topical application for wounds, sedative
Yam - wild	Roots, food, absinthe, topical cream	Phytonutrients (carotene), calcium, iron, magnesium, phosphorous, potassium, selenium, zinc, vitamin Bs	Treatment of muscle spasms, progesterone like
Yerba mate	Leaves, capsules, tincture, tea, beverages	Phytonutrients (caffeine, chlorophyll, Rutin, theobromine etc.), choline, inositol, trace minerals, vitamin Bs C, E	Antioxidant, anti aging, enhances energy, mental focus, appetite suppressant
Yucca	Root, tea, soaps, lotion, powder, tincture	Phytonutrients (beta-carotene, sarsapogenin), calcium, iron, magnesium, manganese, phosphorous, potassium, selenium, zinc, vitamin Bs, C	Anti-inflammatory, anti-arthritic, to treat migraines

NUTRITIONAL DEFICIENCIES

Getting all the nutrients needed solely from food can be a challenge, but it is possible.

However, with soils more deprived of nutrients than ever before, food has fewer nutrients than in the past. Getting adequate nutrients for ideal life and function would require the consumption of much larger quantities of food.

Here are some of the signs and symptoms associated with various deficiencies, along with foods that can help reverse problems. The best way to know if you are deficient in a nutrient is with a blood test by a qualified provider.

SIGNS AND SYMPTOMS OF NUTRITIONAL DEFICIENCIES

Nutrient	Signs & Symptoms of Deficiency	Foods
Biotin	Weak nails and hair, hair loss, muscle loss or weakness, dermatitis	Peanuts, raw egg yolk, dark leafy greens
Boron	Weak bones, arthritis, hormonal imbalance	Apples, oranges, grapes, dates, avocado, beans
Calcium	Muscle cramps and spasms, irritability, insomnia, weak bones and teeth, brittle nails	Dark leafy greens (kale, collard, mustard greens), dairy products
Choline	Weak cell membranes, nerve pain, liver dysfunction	Shrimp, eggs, scallops, chicken turkey, salmon, dark leafy greens
Chromium	Fatigue, irritability, unregulated blood sugar	Green beans, nuts, egg yolk, broccoli, whole grains
Copper	Depression, fatigue, hair loss, weakness	Dark leafy greens, asparagus, squash, nuts and seeds
Essential Fatty Acids	White small bumps on the back of the arms, acne, dandruff, dry skin and hair, eczema, infertility	Seeds, nuts, vegetable oils, cold water fish, flax seed oil, mungo beans
Folic Acid (vitamin B9)	Fatigue, canker sores, tongue patches (geographic tongue), hyperpigmentation, shortness of breath, weakness, diarrhea, forgetfulness	Avocado, spinach, Brussels sprouts, dark leafy greens, nuts, beans, peas, meat, eggs
Iodine	Fatigue, goiter, weight gain	Sea vegetables, scallops, cod, yogurt, shrimp
Iron	Red, enlarged tongue, mouth sores, impaired wound healing, anemia, flattened fingernails	Spinach, dark leafy greens, mulberries, figs
Magnesium	Poor wound healing, irritability, muscle cramps/twitching, weakness, irregular heartbeat	Dark leafy greens, avocadoes, dark chocolate, nuts and seeds
Manganese	Weak joints, muscle loss, weakness, ringing in ears, tremors	Water, whole grains, nuts, vegetables, teas

Niacin (vitamin B3)	Redness at the corners of the mouth, tongue fissures, canker sores, red gums, bad breath, skin inflammation irritability, fatigue, nausea	Fish, peanuts, liver, chicken, fish, whole grains, brewer's yeast
Pantothenic Acid (vitamin B5)	Nausea, muscle spasms, eczema, fatigue, hair loss, irritability, insomnia	Shiitake mushrooms, avocado, sweet potatoes, legumes
Phosphorus	Anxiety, loss of appetite, fatigue, stiff joints, irritability, irregular breathing, weakness	Chard, winter squash, spinach, mushrooms, broccoli
Potassium	Fatigue, acne, muscle weakness, constipation, depression	Beet greens, beans, potatoes, fish, avocado
Riboflavin (vitamin B2)	Redness at the corners of the mouth, gingivitis, inflamed tongue, mouths sores, blurred vision, numbness	Soybeans, spinach, yogurt, mushrooms, beet greens
Selenium	Cold sores, immune problems, increase incidence of cancer	Tuna, shrimps, sardines, salmon, turkey, Brazil nuts
Thiamin (vitamin B1)	Pain sensitivity, nerve pain, weakness, irritability, digestive problems	Sunflower seeds, beans, barley, peas, lentils, oats
Vitamin A	Gingivitis, immune problems, impaired wound healing, fatigue, acne	Sweet potato, carrots, dark leafy greens, squash, liver
Vitamin B6	Impaired wound healing, mouth lesions, loss of hair, nausea, depression	Tuna, meats, salmon, potatoes, sunflower seeds, spinach, banana
Vitamin B12	Fatigue, tongue patches, enlarged tongue, mouth sores, hyperpigmentation, headaches	Sardines, salmon, tuna, scallops, yogurt
Vitamin C	Gingivitis, loose teeth, bruising, cold sores, poor wound healing, infections, fatigue	Papaya, bell pepper, broccoli, Brussels sprouts, strawberries, oranges
Vitamin D	Burning mouth, body aches, muscle cramps, weak bones, impaired healing, infections	Salmon, sardines, tuna, milk, eggs, mushrooms
Vitamin E	Impaired wound healing, nerve problems, immune problems	Sunflower seeds, almonds, avocado, dark leafy greens
Vitamin K	Bruising, bleeding problems, bone weakness, heart disease	Dark leafy greens, parsley, broccoli, Brussels sprouts
Zinc	Tongue patches, impaired wound healing, weak nails, depression, eczema, fatigue	Sesame seeds, pumpkin seeds, lentils, beans, quinoa

As was the case with a patient of mine, Edna, nutritional deficiencies can also intensify pain. Edna suffered from various body aches and joint pain as a result of several deficiencies, ultimately leading to the loss of all her teeth. After we got her nutritional status under control, she underwent a full-mouth rehabilitation with dental implants in one day. Although she reported a slow recovery and pain with her previous dental surgery, she had a remarkable recovery after the implants procedure with minimal pain. Coincidentally, her joint pains and body aches also improved significantly.

In summary, the best way to heal and avoid pain after injury or surgery is by having a healthy body. Just as well, nutrition is the key to achieving that goal.

DIETARY TIPS DURING RECOVERY

1. *Eat a plant-based and low-glycemic diet with an adequate amount of protein.*

2. *Choose colorful fruits and vegetables with as much variety as possible. Colorful fruits and vegetables contain potent antioxidants, which are very important in recovery.*

3. *Eat organic whenever possible. Get familiar with the Dirty Dozen and Clean Fifteen lists by the EPA. The latter of these contain up to 40 percent more antioxidants and have higher levels of minerals and antioxidants.*

4. *Avoid alcoholic beverages, especially prior to any surgery. Excessive alcohol increases inflammation and is a blood thinner.*

5. *Drink plenty of water or herbal tea.*

6. *Chew all food well or use a blender if chewing is difficult.*

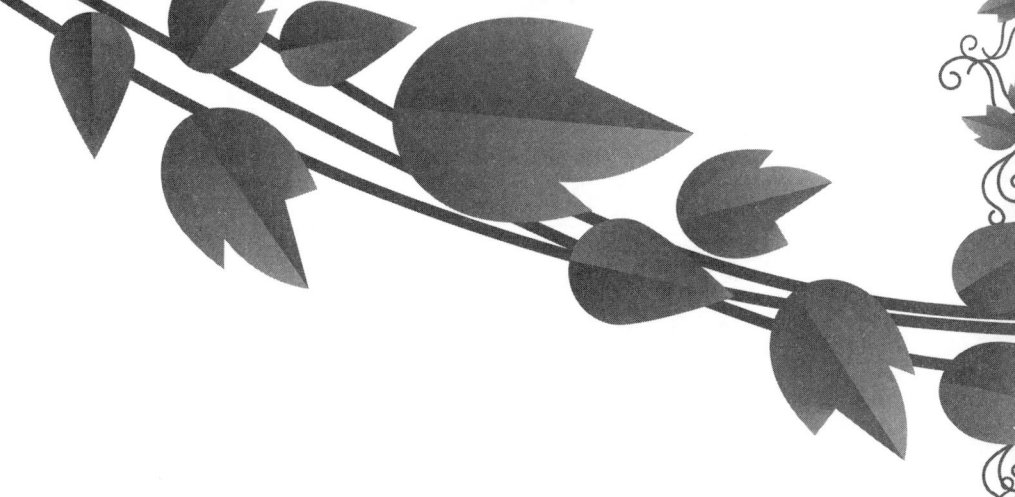

HEALING WITH LIGHT AND ENERGY

I n 2005, my mother was suffering from severe arthritis in her hands. The pain resulting from inflammation was so bad that some days, she couldn't move her joints at all. That same year, I was introduced to Low-Level Laser Therapy (LLLT), which was touted as an option for patients experiencing pain like my mother's.

My first low-level laser was a dual-wavelength, which penetrated about a centimeter into tissue. As soon as I received the machine and was trained on it, I was anxious to try the new methodology on my mother. After using the laser unit for only five minutes, my mother and I were both astounded by the results. The pain level didn't just improve; it vanished! She had immediate relief and she could move her joints freely, without restricted movement or pain.

More and more energetic devices appear on the market, a lot of them for home use. In this chapter, a review of the basis for energy healing will be presented, as well as an overview of different devices which have good success.

BIOENERGETICS—HEALING
THE BODY'S ENERGY

In the world of medicine, there are two competing approaches to the treatment of the human body.

The Newtonian approach basically says that humans are machines, and there are laws that govern how the body acts and reacts to the other forces. Those forces often manifest themselves as sickness and disease, which require other machines (drugs, surgeries, etc.) to correct. Today, medical treatments are dominated by pharmaceutical companies. But drugs come with a price, as evidenced by the long list of possible side effects (including death) rattled off at the end of televised advertisements.

The Einstein approach is the Theory of Relativity, expressed as $E=mc^2$, or energy equals mass multiplied by the speed of light squared. A simple inversion of that formula gets right to the heart of this chapter: all mass is composed of energy. The Einstein approach suggests that humans are not machines, but sums of energy. People are composed of the same material as the rest of the universe.

So, when a human is sick or has a disease, by Einstein's theory, there is an imbalance in that person's energies, which can be corrected with bioenergetics, or energy therapy.

Einstein's work was firmly based in science, and he gave evidence and formulas to communicate what he uniquely understood. While he may have been the first to scientifically connect the dots, he was not the first to conclude that humans are composed of energy, and that the body responds to energy therapies. Those traditions date back to ancient times.

In today's world, it is possible to more fully measure and scientifically describe what it means to have energy disrupted. And there are modern-day advances that harness the healing potential of the most ancient of therapies.

Let me share with you a few energetic devices available today that help promote healing and decrease pain.

LOW-LEVEL LASER THERAPY (LLLT)— HEALING WITH LASERS

Einstein was the first to theorize about lasers in 1906, but it was several decades before people realized the potential of this technology in the world of medicine. The first laser for medicine was presented by Theodor Maiman in 1960. Since then, LLLT has become a very popular treatment used all over the world for ailments ranging from back problems and muscular/skeletal issues, to ulcers, dermatological problems, pain, and swelling. It's also been shown to aid in the body's acceptance of bone transplants, dental implants, and nerve regeneration.[3]

Also known as photobiomodulation, LLLT seems a bit intimidating, conjuring up images of Star Trek warfare or the cutting lasers used in surgery. But LLLT is a painless, cold laser therapy that is

---

3   One study defines LLLT as being "a therapeutic method which regulates the biological behavior of cells with light." It is administered as an external treatment in which the device is placed over the problem area. The laser works by acting on the membranes of the cells in your body, promoting the rapid transport of nutrients in and out of the cells. The laser's energy is transmitted into the cell's internal powerhouse, the mitochondria, which do not function as well during times of stress and injury. Speeding up the activity of the mitochondria helps the cell heal faster. Laser therapy also decreases inflammation and pain by having an effect on the release of the feel-good hormone serotonin, endorphins (neurotransmitters), and bradykinin, which is a blood-dilation compound in the body.

approved by the FDA and has been around for more than three decades. It is not dangerous or harmful, and there are no known side effects.

On the contrary, a laundry list of benefits suggests that LLLT is a powerful tool that can accelerate healing, and the FDA confirms that it can be used for pain relief. More than 2,500 scientific papers have been written on the subject. Including a recent study that found LLLT has positive effects on muscle repair and helps the injured area heal faster, as well as another study showing LLLT promotes tissue repair, inhibits inflammation states, and relieves pain.

The extensive research backing up this therapy was enough to convince me to try it, but my own personal experiences have truly impassioned me. LLLT can be incorporated into treating injuries to the muscle, skin, joint, bone, or as a part of a surgery program to accelerate healing and decrease swelling and pain. Whether the issue is tissue, muscle, implant, sinus, or skeletal related, LLLT can assist in faster healing. Some models for home use can be found on the market, which can be used safely at home.

FOR ONGOING RELIEF

I use LLLT quite often postoperatively to reduce swelling and pain after bone augmentation surgery. It is also beneficial to aid in nerve regeneration for patients who come in with numbness on one side of the lip or tongue. Although the treatment can be used daily, a seven to ten minute session, preferably three to four times a week, is all that it is needed. LLLT also works well for my patients who are just starting to develop a cold sore, or any sore in the mouth for that matter. The light energy can stop ulceration from developing fully, or partially.

Photobiomodulation for wound healing has been extensively studied since 1967. It not only speeds up healing, but also reduces pain. Like my mother, I saw this laser therapy work wonders on a patient, who had oral cancer and was undergoing radiation. She was in so much pain from the mucositis, or inflammation of her mouth due to the radiation, that she could only consume liquids. Mouth sores are quite common in patients undergoing radiation in the face.

Two weeks after using the laser on her ulcers she could eat solid food. Her wounds were on the mend, and her pain was significantly decreased; she was so happy for the relief that she teared up when reporting her progress. Photobiomodulation is the only conventional treatment available for mucositis and paresthesia (nerve damage resulting in numbness).

In dentistry, lasers can be used to accelerate healing after extractions of teeth when dry sockets are present; as well as to decrease sensitivity in a tooth after a composite filling or crown was placed, to heal jaw fractures, and more. Photobiomodulation is also used to treat patients suffering from pain caused by the temporomandibular joint (TMJ), which is located just in front of the ears and connects the lower jaw to the skull. TMJ pain and stiffness can flare up in people with teeth misalignment, missing teeth, or arthritis. One treatment to the jaw relieves pain and relaxes the muscles, allowing the patient to open wide again.

Low-level lasers for home use are available for three to eight thousand dollars. Some combine with light-emitting diodes (LED), while some are LED only, which is not a true laser. LED also has healing potential, but doesn't penetrate as deep.

Although LLLT helps the cells heal and gives effective pain relief, it is not an end-all to treatment. There isn't one. Healing is circular. LLLT is a therapy to be used in conjunction with many other forms of caring to ensure optimal health and the fastest healing possible. For instance, while photobiomodulation will speed up the energy production of the cell, cells still need the right nutrients and water to heal.

LLLT can be used continuously for ongoing relief, even daily. At Beverly Hills Dental Health and Wellness, it is a big part of our post-surgical protocol. But addressing the cause of the pain and discomfort ensures the best and longest-lasting results.

CHROMOTHERAPY—HEALING THROUGH COLOR

I was first exposed to chromotherapy at one of my favorite spas, the Steamboat Healing Center, which has phenomenal geothermal mineral baths and rooms with designated colors.

Chromotherapy, sometimes called color therapy, colorology, or chromatherapy, is the use of colored lights to help your body heal and rebalance itself. Although color is often viewed merely as a backdrop, the colors around us are not randomly prescribed. Each color is an actual form of energy—a fact that can be scientifically proven.

Science shows different frequencies manifest themselves as different colors of light. Each frequency is unique and affects the body in different ways: mentally, physically, emotionally, and, some would argue, even spiritually.

The organs and different parts of the body are composed of their own colors, which in turn indicate a unique frequency. A disruption to those frequencies causes an imbalance to the body, allowing disease or other physical malfunctions to set in. The effects manifest themselves in physical, emotional, and mental health.

Chromotherapy exposes the body to the exact frequency needed to return harmony and allow it to self-balance and heal. For example, someone suffering with diabetes would be exposed to yellow light, which is the color of the pancreas. Yellow light is considered a laxative and diuretic, which stimulates the brain, liver, and spleen.

A study published in 2005 found that: "When applied to the human body, light will provide all deficient energies since every color is associated with a quantity of energy." However, some researchers argue that the light is first transmitted to the electromagnetic field, or aura, surrounding our bodies—which can be scientifically measured, even though it can't be seen—and that field then delivers the healing energies.

Color therapy is often tightly associated to the idea that our body has seven different energy centers, or chakras, each associated with a specific color of visible light.

The color theories date back to ancient Egypt, Greece, China, and India, with the use of color therapy being recorded as early as 2000 B.C. The practitioners at that time may not have had a full understanding of the science behind the outcomes they observed, but they were definitely sold on "color medicine."

The following chart details how each color can be used to accelerate healing.

THE COLOR CHART

Color	What It Does	Diseases Affected
Red	Activates the circulatory and nervous systems, spine, and pelvic area.	Blood disorders, anemias
Strong Pink	Acts as a cleanser, strengthens the veins and arteries.	Blood disorders, anemias
Pink	Activates and eliminates impurities from the blood stream.	Blood disorders, anemias
Orange	Energizes intestinal area, kidneys, and bladder. Helps address asthma and bronchitis.	Obesity, disorders of lungs, and kidneys
Strong Yellow	Strengthens the body and acts on internal issues.	Immune problems
Yellow	Reactivates and purifies the skin. Helps with digestion and physical stress.	Disorders of stomach, pancreas, and liver
Green	Acts as a relaxant. Promotes tissue regeneration.	Heart disease and hypertension
Strong Green	Provides anti-infectious, antiseptic, and regenerative stimulation.	Infections, injuries
Strong Blue	Lubricates joints. Helps address infections, stress, and nervous tension.	Joint injuries, stress, infections
Blue	Stimulates muscle and skin cells, nerves, and the circulatory system. Increases oxygen.	Muscle and skin injuries, cuts, throat-related issues
Indigo	Helps address eye inflammation, cataracts, glaucoma. and ocular fatigue.	Disorders of the eye
Violet	Relaxes the nerves and lymphatic system. Anti-inflammatory and energizing.	Inflammatory problems, stress, anxiety

Sources: Richard Gerber M.D., *Vibrational Medicine: the #1 handbook of subtle-energy therapies*, (Rochester: Bear & Company, 2001).

SUNLIGHT—THE PERFECT BLEND

Sunlight is the perfect blend of all seven visible colors. Its health benefits are underappreciated in today's society, where we are quick to cover ourselves in long sleeves and sunblock in order to keep the sun at bay.

But the sun can revitalize, protect from disease, and synchronize hormonal rhythms. Just as a flower cannot grow in the darkness, the human body also needs sunlight for optimal health.

Stepping into the sunlight has almost an immediate effect. Since the body is electrically charged, the sun provides immediate rejuvenation. It has a calming effect on the brain, and regulates hormonal rhythm. For example, melatonin, a powerful antioxidant that helps to regulate sleep patterns, is heavily affected by light and dark. The lack of sunlight can affect the regulation of this hormone and lead to sleep issues.

In areas where there are fewer days of sunshine annually, such as in the Pacific Northwest, there is a higher overall rate of depression due to Seasonal Affective Disorder, which stems from a lack of sunlight. The remedy is sunshine, which some get from full-spectrum lights that mimic the sun's rays.

The sun is also the most abundant and natural source of vitamin D, an important component of good health. Studies have shown a correlation between a vitamin D deficiency, and higher rates of illness and infections. Vitamin D is also key to bone healing and calcium absorption from food. And yet, more people are taking vitamin D supplements, especially people who tend to get sick more often. But why pop a pill when you can step into the sunlight and soak it in yourself? Dr. Mercola, a renowned expert on health, says, "I am beyond convinced that you are missing the boat on vitamin D big time if you merely rely on swallowing pills or capsules."

I have seen first-hand the problems with vitamin D. For instance, in spite of impeccable oral hygiene, Maria, a patient of mine, had recurring infections and several episodes of colds and bronchitis following a dental implant that was done with augmented bone. It turned out she had very low vitamin D; once that level was raised via supplementation, her infections ceased. It took three months of oral supplementation to raise her levels from 19 to 50 ng/ml (nanograms/ milliliter); 50 ng/ml is the level recommended by the Vitamin D Council. Another patient, who moved to Southern California from Seattle for health reasons, had lingering fatigue, depression, and lung issues, such as recurring flu, colds, and bronchitis. After her vitamin D levels rose following repeated exposure to the California sun and oral supplementation, she was able to get her energy back and keep the flu away. Her periodontal disease, which I was treating her for, also improved significantly. More on Vitamin D testing and supplementation in Chapter 7.

EARTHING—GETTING GROUNDED

Have you noticed that people coming back from vacation usually look and feel better? It's because they literally are better. The contact they've had with the earth as they spent time on the beach or hiking with the family physically rejuvenates them in measurable ways. The exact term for this phenomenon is called earthing, or grounding.

Earthing may be a new term to you, but it is a simple principle that can be easily applied to your life. Earthing involves going outside and connecting with the earth—literally. Research in earthing is still ongoing, but what we know so far is that earthing improves sleep, energy, blood pressure; lowers stress, muscle tension, inflammation, and chronic pain, while most importantly, accelerating healing.

Clint Ober has done a lot of research in the field of earthing. His work has helped reveal that it is possible to reconnect to the Earth's healing energy. Because the body is basically a complex electrical circuit, electricity regulates the flow of nutrients in and out of the body's cells. The nervous system, muscles, and literally every organ, including the heart, are bioelectrical systems.

In fact, other studies have shown that direct contact with the earth (hiking barefoot, hugging a tree, gardening) can actually neutralize unhealthy positive charges the body develops by picking up a negative charge through free electrons from the earth. Dr. Joseph Mercola says that, "(T)hese free electrons are probably the most potent antioxidants known to man. These antioxidants are responsible for the clinical observations from grounding experiments, such as beneficial changes in heart rate, decreased skin resistance, (and) decreased levels of inflammation."

Stress, injury, working indoors, and consumption of processed foods adds positive charges to the body throughout the day, which alter the body's electric field leading to depression. Higher levels of depression are usually seen in people that do little to no earthing, such as those who live in high rises or rainy cities.

Earthing can help your body repair itself faster, and keep you more comfortable after an injury by protecting you from inflammation. Research shows that grounding, or earthing, after an injury, infuses your body and tissues with electrons, which immediately neutralizes the harmful free radicals. Research conducted on cyclists found that those who grounded after their daily race reported almost zero tendonitis and faster healing of injuries. Today, many top athletes, such as triathletes, NFL players, and swimmers, use earthing.

Luckily, it's easy to repair the body's electrical field and bring it back into balance. Simply tossing off your shoes and taking a quick stroll around the yard or in a park gives you an immediate connection to the earth. Walking barefoot is one of the easiest and most effective ways to do earthing, because the body's most powerful conductor—the kidney point—is located on the ball of the foot. There is a similar point in your hand. There are whole communities in places like Austria, Switzerland, and Germany, which maintain a tradition of walking around barefoot first thing in the morning. What a great way to start the day!

There is no exact prescription or methodology for earthing. The key is to just do it, and for at least thirty minutes at a time: constantly connect with the earth in order to maintain that favorable electrical charge.

One of the best places to spend time outdoors is on the beach, since seawater is considered one of the best conductors. Earthing on other water sources—even dewy grass—may increase your body's ability to conduct its electrons more effectively. Concrete is also a good conductor, but only if it hasn't been painted or sealed.

Asphalt, wood, plastic, and the soles of your shoes can inhibit the flow of electrons. However, some shoe products are made with earthing in mind.

You may know that electricians wear rubber-soled shoes for their protection because they block the electric current from the earth. Without those shoes, then connecting to a dangerous electric current would be magnified, because it would ground them to the powerful electric source coming from the earth.

Rubber shoes are crucial when working with electricity, but for the rest of us—and for the rest of your life—toss the rubber shoes and *connect* with the earth. You don't want to block that powerful life force from coming into your body to keep you balanced and accelerate your healing.

HEALING WITH MICROCURRENT THERAPY

As scientists began to explore the effect of different frequencies of microcurrents on the body, so did the study of the body's natural electrical current. Microcurrent therapy was first used in Europe in the 1980s to stimulate bone repair in non-union fractures.

Today, microcurrent therapy is growing in popularity as an alternative option for helping injured tissue heal faster and providing relief from injury or chronic conditions, decreasing the need for medication.

Microcurrent therapy works because it raises cellular energy by up to 500 percent, which increases the rate of healing in wounds and fractures. In his book, *The Body Electric: Electromagnetism and the Foundation of Life*, Robert Becker, MD, describes how the body's cells cannot do their job efficiently without the proper electromagnetic signals. The body's natural electrical current allows communication between cells; that electrical current is disturbed when an area is injured, whether intentionally or unintentionally. Microcurrent also increases nutrient transport into the cell by 70 percent. It also removes toxins, increases circulation, and has been proven effective on non-healing ulcers. Clinically, it was observed that wounds close 45 percent faster when microcurrent therapy is used postsurgically.

Microcurrent differs from conventional electrical stimulation, in that the current delivered is a thousand times less intense. The treatment is safe and painless, although a slight tingling can be felt where the very low-voltage current comes in contact with the surface of the skin. The treatment lasts from five to thirty minutes, depending on the condition being treated. There are no adverse side effects. However, it is contraindicated in people who have pacemakers, and should be avoided during pregnancy. For best results, hydration is key prior to undergoing treatment.

RESULTS IN MINUTES

In my practice, I use microcurrent therapy daily to relieve post-surgical pain and swelling, and to treat TMJ discomfort. Usually, I see results within minutes, although chronic conditions may take several visits to resolve. Today, microcurrent devices can be purchased for home use, and are small enough to take when traveling. Practitioners combining microcurrent therapy with color light therapy and sound healing methods have found that they work synergistically to accelerate healing of the connective tissue, muscles, nerves, brain cells, and other organs. Microlight therapy, as it is called, was first described in 2002. Microlight works for pain relief, aesthetic, and emotional healing, as well as rehabilitation from injuries, strokes, and neurodegenerative diseases.

Microcurrent and microlight work similar to acupuncture, by clearing stagnation and increasing the flow of energy. Since there are no side effects with either, I highly recommend you give these a try in lieu of prescription medications, which have numerous side effects.

A WORD ABOUT ACUPUNCTURE

Microcurrent is sometimes used in conjunction with acupuncture. The needles are connected to electrodes, and a low level of electricity is transmitted into the skin.

Acupuncture is the most well known and widely studied of all the energy-based therapies. Acupuncture involves the insertion of very fine needles into specific points on the energetic meridians of the body where vital life energy flows. I have had acupuncture many times with great results, whether it was for tendonitis in my hand, lack of energy, or a bad cold.

Acupuncture originated in China thousands of years ago, but its popularity has grown worldwide in the past three decades. A national survey in 2007 estimated that over three million people in the United States have used acupuncture. That figure was expected to increase every year as more people seek out alternatives to conventional medicine, especially for pain management.

While pain is one of the primary reasons people seek treatment using acupuncture, the treatment has been found to offer relief for a wide range of issues. Among these is fibromyalgia, a debilitating condition that manifests itself in joint and muscle pain. In fact, a 2006 Mayo Clinic study found that acupuncture significantly improved the symptoms of fibromyalgia, which has no treatment in conventional medicine except for pain medication. Studies also show that acupuncture works on headaches and migraines, with relief experienced after a twenty-minute treatment.

It is also a great addition to many conventional treatments, such as chemotherapy and cardiac surgery. The Mayo Clinic found that acupuncture significantly reduced nausea, vomiting, and overall discomfort in patients pre and posttreatment. Research has also shown acupunc-

COMMON CONDITIONS TREATED WITH MICROCURRENT THERAPY:

- Arthritis
- Back pain
- Bone fractures
- Fibromyalgia
- Frozen shoulder
- Headaches
- Inflammation—chronic and acute
- Joint pain
- Muscular problems
- Nerve injuries
- Postsurgical pain and swelling
- Scar tissue
- Sports injuries
- TMJ pain
- Wound healing

ture can help the body protect against infections by raising white blood-cell count, which are responsible for the immune system.

A number of studies have also shown the effectiveness of acupuncture pain from a dental abscess or oral surgery.

Acupuncture may be combined with conventional treatments to control the pain and reduce the amount of medication needed following surgery.

Most importantly, acupuncture has proven to be a safe therapy. The World Health Organization (WHO) and the National Institutes of Health (NIH) found it to be an effective treatment for many different mental, physical, and spiritual health conditions.

Acupuncture is a proven treatment for:

- Adverse reactions to radiotherapy and/or chemotherapy
- Allergic rhinitis (including hay fever)
- Biliary colic
- Depression (including depressive neurosis and depression following stroke)
- Dysentery, acute bacillary
- Dysmenorrhoea, primary
- Epigastralgia, acute (in peptic ulcer, acute and chronic gastritis, and gastrospasm)
- Facial pain (including craniomandibular disorders)
- Headache
- Hypertension, essential
- Hypotension, primary
- Induction of labor
- Knee pain
- Leukopenia
- Low back pain
- Malposition of fetus, correction of morning sickness
- Nausea and vomiting
- Neck pain
- Pain in dentistry (including dental pain and temporomandibular dysfunction)

- Periarthritis of shoulder

- Postoperative pain

- Renal colic

- Rheumatoid arthritis

- Sciatica Sprain

- Stroke

- Tennis elbow

Sources: World Health Organization and National Institutes of Health

PULSED ELECTROMAGNETIC FIELD THERAPY (PEMF)—RENEWING ENERGY

Pulsed Electromagnetic Field Therapy (PEMF) has been widely used in Western Europe for some time. The first reported use of electromagnetic current for bone healing occurred in 1841. But its use in North America did not start until 1979, when the FDA approved the first device for stimulating bone growth in non-healing bone fractures. That occurred after Andrew Bassett, MD, demonstrated in 1974 that a pulsed magnetic field applied across the side of a bone fracture accelerates the healing process.

Now, you may have heard about how detrimental electromagnetic fields are to the human body. Computers, power lines, televisions, Wi-Fi, cellphones, and other technologies have an electromagnetic field, which can actually interfere with that of the human body. Those energies are draining because they are a much different frequency than the electromagnetic field occurring within nature and the human body. Some people are actually more sensitive to the electromagnetic fields of electronics.

But PEMF (sometimes abbreviated as PEMFT) has different frequencies that resemble those produced by the body. Every organ has its own signature electromagnetic frequency, which controls the biochemical reactions that go on inside and between the body's cells. If a healthy electromagnetic field in the body is disrupted by an external field, then cellular dysfunction and ultimately disease can result.

PEMF treatment can restore the body's healthy electromagnetic field. Used alone or in conjunction with other treatments, it has been shown to reduce pain and inflammation, while improving energy, circulation, and the uptake of nutrients into the cell. It accelerates the repair of bone, muscles, connective tissue, and skin. It can also calm a hyperactive immune system, or stimulate a failing one.

The device does not touch the skin. Instead, it hovers over the area being treated and pulses electromagnetic field through the body to restore the electrical circuit. Treatment can last from five to thirty minutes, but its effect can last for hours or days. It is usually given once or twice a day, for two or more weeks. William Pawluk, MD, a major advocate of PEMF therapy, says that PEMF is regularly needed to help tune up cells and keep them healthy.

The FDA approved PEMF treatment for depression in 2011, for people who did not respond well to antidepressant medication. Antidepressants have horrible side effects, including dry mouth, which can result in thousands of dollars in dental work. PEMF treatment of the head for depression, also called transcranial magnetic stimulation (TMS), has no side effects. The method used stimulates small regions of the brain. TMS is also useful for neuropathic pain, and evaluating damage from a range of neuromuscular diseases and disorders affecting the face.

When seeking treatment from a health practitioner for PEMF therapy, look for one who is experienced in using the devices.

Handheld PEMF devices can also be purchased for home use, and they are relatively easy to operate and sometimes come with a tutorial. In my opinion, every household should have a microcurrent/PEMF device. They are helpful for dealing with trauma, daily stress, or the inability to fall asleep. I believe we will see more of these devices being used, since they are also great anti-aging tools.

Infoceuticals—Drops of Energy

Peter Fraser, an Australian professor of acupuncture in Chinese medicine, researched the human body field, another term for the body's electromagnetic field, for more than twenty years. The body field is a network of information and energy that helps coordinate all of the body's physiological functions.

Fraser correlated quantum physics to the body's energy meridians to explain, for the first time, a comprehensive view of the energetic field surrounding the human body and its relationship to physiological functions. Fraser found a way to correct distortions in the body field caused by environmental stresses, poor diet, and external electromagnetic fields, so that the body may return to its normal state of health. His lifelong research has been put into practice around the world, allowing health practitioners to scan the human body field and provide the right treatment to the area experiencing distortions.

Fraser's treatment consists of microcurrent/PEMF therapy along with energetic drops, called infoceuticals, which are minerals infused with different energetic frequencies in an alcohol suspension.

Although the technology is still in its infancy, I have experienced amazing results with my own health and with patients.

Take Michael, for instance, who came to see me because of an acute and persistent mouth infection, and an overall feeling of unwellness that had lingered following a viral infection ten months prior. Using the energetic scan by NES ProHealth, I prescribed Michael a series of infoceuticals in conjunction with treating his oral infection. After the first treatment, Michael felt life returning to his body. Three months later, he was fully back to normal and his oral infection was resolved.

THE ROLE OF ENERGY IN HEALING

Ignoring the new and emerging field of bioenergetics in medicine is simply not possible anymore. Although modern medicine has a role in treating disease, pharmaceutical medications are making people sicker than ever. Now is the time to recognize that we are energetic beings. The human body's electrical circuit must be maintained in order to achieve optimum health and healing. Thoughts also have an energetic effect on cellular health. The next chapter explores ways to influence healing based on thoughts and behavior.

....

CHAPTER 4

HEALING WITH MEDITATION, GUIDED IMAGERY, AND SLEEP

P art of the reason healing of the body and mind can be difficult after a surgical procedure or injury, is because of the stress involved. Stress is the mind's perception in relation to an event that is happening or that is about to happen. When it comes to surgery, the perceived pain and swelling following the procedure causes stress, which in turn, increases pain and swelling. It's a vicious cycle largely brought on by cortisol, which is known as "the stress hormone."

Cortisol is released during periods of fear and stress, and is known to slow down healing and weaken the immune system. Inadequate or excessive production of cortisol by the adrenal glands in response to stress can eventually lead to imbalances in blood glucose levels, impaired immune response, and a host of different hormonal imbalances. All of which are associated with multiple adverse conditions and symptoms.

As a student at Ohio State University, I witnessed research on wound healing. The study involved a pea-sized wound being created on the roof of the mouth of dental students during vacation time and then right before finals to compare rates of healing. The results clearly show that during finals, wound healing slowed significantly. Many other studies in medicine have shown that mental stress delays healing, but that relaxation can accelerate the healing. After all, our thoughts do influence physical changes in our body.

In fact, it is now scientifically proven that our thoughts can change the brain. Images of the brain during meditation show physical changes happen at a cellular level. The mind and body are wired together through the central nervous system, and there is constant two-way communication between the mind and the body, both conscious and unconscious. This allows for a "rewiring" of the brain, which is known as neuroplasticity. Rewiring your brain can improve healing and your overall well-being. Research has shown that even the adult brain can change, from microscopic changes in neurons (cells in your brain excited by your body's electrical and chemical signals) to cortical remapping in response to injury.

TESTING FOR CORTISOL

If you are feeling stressed, and wondering whether your cortisol levels are out of balance, consider having your cortisol levels tested. Cortisol levels can be assessed in the saliva, blood, or urine; saliva or urine are more accurate than blood measurements. Ask your doctor to conduct this test prior to any surgery. Some labs may be contacted directly to request a saliva kit test come to your house. If your levels are especially high, you should postpone your surgery until the levels were decreased within normal range.

Cortical remapping is reorganizing the way your brain responds to sensory input. For instance, when you touch something with your hand, it sends a signal to your brain. Neuroplastic change can be caused by learning a new task, a different way of thinking, or through different experiences and activities, such as meditation and exercise.

Learning to cope with fear and stress are important in any situation, but especially during healing. There are a number of easy-to-follow techniques for coping with fear and stress. By learning techniques for deep relaxation, you can experience less pain after surgery or recovering from an injury. These techniques may lower the risk of infection and the degree of complications. Once you notice they're benefits, you will want to continue these on a daily basis.

Meditation—It's About Focus

Meditation comes from Eastern spiritual traditions and has been practiced for thousands of years. Recently, however, meditation has been on the rise. The University of California, Los Angeles (UCLA), has implemented the Mindful Awareness Research Center, which offers classes to strengthen meditation practices.

Contrary to what some believe, meditation is not clearing the mind by thinking about nothing. During meditation, it is important to focus on something. Breathing is focused during meditation, and often chanting (the repetition of a word, sound, or phrase) is used. Chanting helps keep the mind focused on the meditation.

TYPES OF MEDITATION

- Primordial sound meditation (PSM) is a silent way of practicing and uses a vibrational sound called "mantra."

- Mindfulness-based stress reduction (MBSR) uses the breathing and focuses attention on the body.

- Analytical meditation focuses on the object and trying to understand the deeper meaning.

- Breath or zen meditation uses the connection between the breath and the mind in a seated position.

- Mindfulness meditation is about having increased awareness about how you feel at that moment.

- Transcendental meditation is a seated type of meditation using a mantra spoken out loud or silently.

- Walking or moving meditation focuses the attention on the soles of your feet as you are walking or dancing.

To better understand the techniques of meditation when just starting out, it is helpful to join a class or consult a teacher.

PRACTICING MINDFULNESS MEDITATION

Mindfulness is being present, focusing and accepting the way you feel now, acknowledging your thoughts and emotions in the present. According to a recent issue of *Science*, mindfulness can impact different conditions. It reduces stress and chronic physical pain, while boosting the immune system, positive emotions, and inducing a state of well-being. Research also shows that mindfulness has a positive effect on not only pain and anxiety, but also psoriasis and the immune function.

Professor of Medicine Emeritus, Jon Kabat-Zinn, developed a mindfulness-based stress reduction program (MBSR). His technique combines meditation with a branch of yoga known as Hatha. His first book, *Full Catastrophe Living: Using the Wisdom of Your Body and Mind to Face Stress, Pain, and Illness*, gives a description of his technique. While practicing yoga and studying with Buddhist teachers, he realized that he must help others integrate these teachings in everyday life to help them cope with stress, anxiety, pain, and diseases. He opened the first mindfulness center in the United States, in 1979, at the University of Massachusetts medical school. The program Kabat-Zinn created is now used by other medical centers and hospitals across the country.

I have been practicing mindfulness meditation for several years now. Here are a few tips for mindfulness meditation:

- Find a comfortable position either on a chair or with your back against the wall.

- If you are flexible enough to cross your legs, go ahead, but it is not necessary to do so.

- Start breathing from the abdomen and monitor your breath as it goes in and out through the nose.

- As your mind wanders away from the breath, bring your awareness back to the breath.

When starting mindfulness meditation, begin with at least ten-minute sessions. With practice it will become easier to meditate for longer periods of time.

Compared to medications such as Xanax and Ambien, which are addictive yet commonly used for anxiety and sleep, meditation is a great alternative with no side effects. Throw away those pills and try meditation. You will not regret it.

HEALING THROUGH HYPNOSIS
AND GUIDED IMAGERY

Hypnosis is the induction of an altered state of perception and memory, elicited by suggestion. The mind is literally put in a trance, almost like daydreaming.

Hypnosis comes from the Greek word *hypnos*, which means "sleep." The application of hypnosis to alter pain and state of mind dates back centuries. A German physician considered to be the founder of western hypnotherapy, Franz Mesmer, believed that an illness is caused by an imbalance in the magnetic fluids of the body and that the transfer of magnetism from the hypnotist to the individual could correct the imbalance.

Functional neuroimaging studies support the clinical use of hypnosis in the management of pain conditions. The Mayo Clinic also reports that hypnosis helps lower anxiety prior to medical or dental procedures, and the effect can last for up to three years. Furthermore, the National Institutes of Health also endorses the evidence that shows the effectiveness of this technique treating pain associated with cancer, fibromyalgia, TMJ disorders, and dental procedures.

Today, some practitioners use hypnosis at the time of conscious sedation for minor surgical cases and have reported positive results. Medical research has also looked at hypnosis for severe and persistent pain relief. According to one study, a preoperative hypnosis session can significantly reduce the need for pain medication after surgical removal of wisdom teeth. Another study found that hypnosis significantly reduced the nausea and vomiting following general anesthesia in a group of women who listened to audio tapes for four to six days prior to surgery.

Although studies are limited when looking at the rate of healing postsurgically, Carol Ginandes, PhD, published some great research on the subject. She demonstrated that incisions heal at a faster rate when hypnosis is used. When comparing bone fracture X-rays after six weeks of healing, the patients practicing hypnotherapy healed faster.

Traditionally, hypnosis consists of three stages: pre-suggestion, suggestion, and post-suggestion. Here are some examples of hypnotic suggestions:

- "When you're done with the surgery, you will feel happy and free of all pain."
- "You are healing at a rapid pace, free of pain."
- "The broken bone is getting stronger each day and you will be back on your feet within days."
- "The incision is closing rapidly without a scar."

Guided imagery may also be considered a form of hypnotherapy. Guided imagery is a technique using soothing mental imagery to help heal anything from a small wound to a surgical incision or even cancer. It has been scientifically studied to reduce stress and promote healing, and is often used to treat pain, chronic or acute. Evidence even shows that it can reduce the side effects of chemotherapy. The technique can also be used ahead of surgery to help reduce stress and fear; patients heal faster listening to hypnotically delivered suggestions prior to surgery.

Guided imagery is not a new technique. It was a practiced in ancient Greece, where it was believed that strong images of disease can actually cause symptoms. The Navajo Indians also have guided imagery in their culture, encouraging a person to see him or herself as "healthy." The father of psychoanalysis, Sigmund Freud, and renowned psychiatrist, Carl Jung, also documented curing diseases with the imagination.

The Mayo Clinic endorses guided imagery, and researchers have found that guided imagery influences specific physical changes. Brain PET (positron emission tomography) scans visually show which part of the brain is being activated during guided imagery. Guided imagery can increase white blood cells to fortify the immune system. The treatment has a direct effect on heart and respiration rates, as well as blood pressure.

When a patient has high blood pressure prior to a dental procedure in my office, which is usually caused by stress or a perception of pain over the course of the procedure, I often use guided imagery to help lower it. By helping the mind focus on soothing images, the whole body can relax, which can lower the blood pressure. I normally see a drop in the patient's blood pressure within ten minutes of using the technique. Practicing guided imagery two to four times before surgery helps reduce fear and anxiety, and decreases the need for medication after the procedure. Those who use guided imagery are commonly discharged from the hospital one or two days earlier than those who do not use it.

HOW TO PRACTICE GUIDED IMAGERY

The easiest way to practice guided imagery is by listening to an audio file during recovery. But guided imagery can also be practiced with a hypnotherapist or a psychiatrist. Suggestions, together with effective breathing and relaxing, are given in the course of treatment. As the session progresses, a solution to the patient's problem is presented.

Marc Schoen, author of *Your Survival Instinct is Killing You*, has specialized in mind-body medicine for more than twenty-five years. He currently teaches medical students at UCLA about the role of the mind in health. He has developed techniques called Hypno-Conditioning, which combine hypnosis with mind-conditioning. In researching these techniques, he found them to be particularly effective in helping treat headaches, pain, stress, arthritis, postsurgical recovery, skin disorders, and intestinal inflammation. He has created audio files for different conditions, one of them specifically for postsurgical healing. I have personally used the files and can attest to their effectiveness. The deep sleep hypnosis file is so effective that I can never get to the end of it without falling to sleep.

Peggy Huddleston has also developed a mind-body program to help recovery after surgery. Using her techniques, people feel calmer before surgery, use 23 to 50 percent less pain medication, and recover faster. She describes her five-step technique in her book *Prepare for Surgery, Heal Faster:*

Step one: Relax while listening to the CD provided with her program.

Step two: Visualize your recovery by turning fears into healing images.

Step three: Organize a support group to help you hear loving thoughts from your friends and family.

Step four: Use healing statements. These are given to the surgeon or nurse to say during surgery.

Step five: Meet the anesthesiologist before the day of the surgery.

For more information on Huddleston's process to prepare for surgery, visit her website, www.healfaster.com.

In her book, Huddleston gives examples and scientific research that affirmation during surgery can affect a patient's recovery. When someone is under sedation, their consciousness is still aware of the surroundings.

In my practice, conscious sedation is performed by an anesthesiologist for longer procedures involving full-mouth rehabilitation with dental implants. We use conscious sedation instead of general anesthesia because swallowing and other reflexes are kept intact. If I feel a patient is agitated, I always reassure them that everything is going great and they will recover fast. It seems to have a calming effect, not just on the patient, but also on me. When I feel my patient stressing out, I can get stressed out as well, so the calming effect helps us both.

That is universally true of all health practitioners: We feel the stress of our patients. One of my patients actually asked me to join in a prayer with her at the beginning of her procedure. Prayer is a form of visualization healing, and part of the mind-body connection.

When first trying guided imagery, I highly recommend using an audio file as a guide, or receiving counseling over the phone or in person on how to complete the technique. After the first few tries, you'll be able to do it by yourself. Here are a few tips:

- Find an area where you can relax without distractions. If you're in the hospital, consider using earplugs.

- Begin with slow, deep breaths; on the exhale, release all tension and negative thoughts.

- Focus on breathing through the belly button and feel your stomach rise and fall with every breath.

- Now, find an image that makes you happy. It could be a beautiful beach in Hawaii, or the face of a loved one. Focus on this image while breathing slowly.

- Combine the image with a positive sentence or word. For example, if you're imagining a beautiful beach in Hawaii, say to yourself, "I feel relaxed and at peace."

The question I hear most often about hypnosis is: "Am I able to be hypnotized?" That is a great question. The best answer I can give comes from a quote by Henry Ford: "If you think you can or think you can't, either way you're right." That means it's all up to you. If you don't want to be hypnotized, you simply won't get to experience it. However, if you're open to hypnosis and you are receptive to it, then you will get good results.

THE ROLE OF SLEEP IN HEALING

The pace of life has changed greatly in the last fifty years. Take, for example, a busy day in New York City: It starts with running from home to get coffee, then to work, then to an appointment, and finally back home or out to dinner. All of these things are being done at the expense of sleep. A recent study by the National Institutes of Health revealed that, these days, an adult in the United States gets less than seven hours of sleep nightly, compared to eight and a half hours in 1960, and roughly one-third of adults sleep less than six hours per night.

Many of my patients are sleep deprived. Those who are always on the run and lack sleep have the poorest healing. By that I mean, because of their slow-healing wounds, they are in more pain than most and the mucosa, or moist tissue, appears to recover more slowly. So how does sleep affect a person's healing?

The body repairs and renews during sleep. A body healing from surgery or injury needs more rest and sleep, because the body needs more energy directed to the affected area; leaving less for other activities. Studies have even shown that lack of sleep exacerbates pain following surgery or injury.

If you are someone who thinks you can survive, and even thrive, without sleep, think again. Nothing can replace a good night's sleep when it comes to your health: no medication or treatment. Sleep deprivation can have serious effects on healing. Markers in the body that signal inflammation, such as C-reactive protein (CRP), increase. The risks of autoimmune diseases, high blood pressure, and vascular diseases also increase when inflammation markers are high. Have you noticed that you are more irritable when you don't get enough sleep? That's because lack of sleep leads to less tolerance of things—like pain.

Optimally, adults need seven to nine hours of sleep per night. During that time, a person will go through several cycles of the five stages of sleep.

Stage one is a transition between being awake and being asleep. Some muscle activity and movement still exist in this stage.

Stage two is when heart rate begins to decrease and the body temperature drops.

Stage three is a deep sleep, also called restorative sleep. It is the most important sleep during healing. In stage three, the brain enters the delta waves state.

Stage four is a deeper restorative sleep when the body's ability to regenerate increases. The body is working on rebuilding its forces, including the immune system. The production of certain growth hormones also increase, contributing the regeneration of different cells during healing.

Stage five, or REM (rapid eye movement), is the dreaming stage. REM occurs right before waking.

SLEEP APNEA

Many patients go undiagnosed with what is ultimately a very dangerous condition. Most people don't realize the repercussions of sleep apnea. It can lead to high blood pressure, increased risk of cardiovascular disease, diabetes, ADHD, and a shorter lifespan.

One of my patients, Maria, is evidence of the connection between sleep apnea and cardiovascular disease. In her mid-seventies, Maria started developing atrial fibrillations, or an abnormal heart rhythm. Her cardiologist encouraged her to get a sleep test, which found that she had moderate sleep apnea. A dental sleep apnea appliance

> ### TIPS FOR A GOOD SLEEP:
>
> - No caffeine past one o'clock in the afternoon
> - Keep your cellphone away from your bed
> - No electronic devices within ten feet of your bed
> - No tight clothing/ pajamas
> - Complete deep breathing exercises or meditation for at least five minutes before sleep
> - Enjoy a cup of chamomile or lavender/ valerian tea

was made for her at our office, which helped her reposition her jaw forward so that more oxygen would go into her lungs when breathing at night. Overtime, her atrial fibrillations diminished significantly.

Apnea is a complete cessation (stoppage) of breathing for at least ten seconds; hypopnea is when the breath is constricted for more than ten seconds. The total episodes of apnea and hypopnea in an hour gives an index number, which then allows the doctor to categorize mild, moderate, or severe conditions of sleep apnea.

I highly recommend getting a sleep test for sleep apnea. In the past, testing for sleep apnea required the patient to go to a sleep lab and spend the night in a cold, uncomfortable room. Modern technology allows the test to take place in the comfort of your home simply by wearing a strapped-on monitor. There is also a comfortable T-shirt that monitors breathing patterns and oxygen saturation while sleeping.

People who should get tested for sleep apnea include those who:

- Snore loudly
- Frequently wake during sleep
- Have high blood pressure
- Are overweight
- Can't stay awake during the day

A lack of sleep can also dysregulate certain genes that give rise to tumors. The World Health Organization calls lack of sleep a human carcinogen.

So, meditation, guided imagery, and proper sleep can help improve overall health and promote better healing. What the body needs most, however, is oxygen.

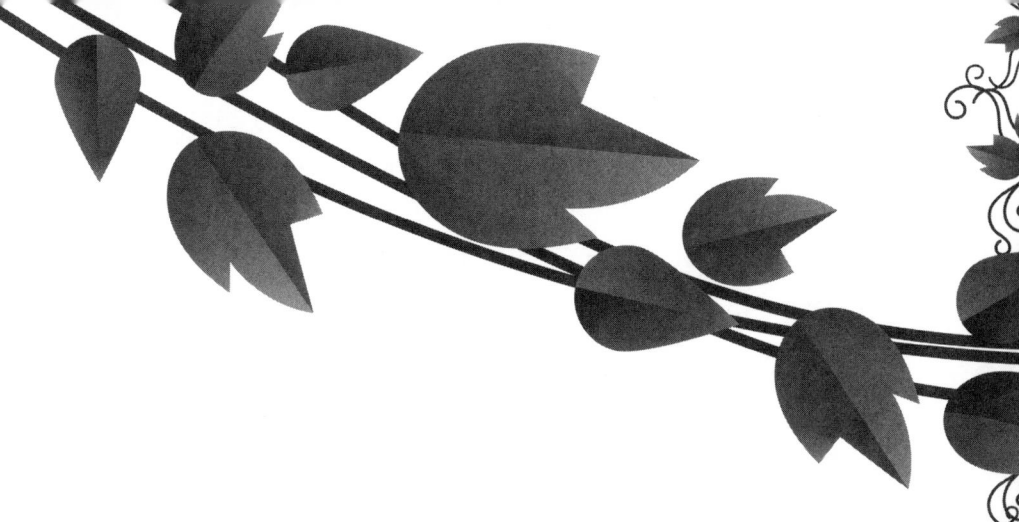

···

CHAPTER 5

HEALING WITH OXYGEN

B ack in 2006, I was involved in a diving accident in which I inhaled water about sixty feet under the surface. Fortunately, I survived to tell that story. But it affected me in my daily life in ways I could never have imagined. For a long time, I couldn't get in an elevator; it was hard for me to fly.

What I would learn with the help of cognitive therapy was that my brain was falsely telling me I didn't have enough air in tight spaces. My trained cognitive therapist guided me through three stages of acknowledgement that put me on the path to recovery. The first stage was to identify the "activating agent," or the source of the problem. In my case, it was the diving accident. The second stage was to focus on the "belief" I was laboring under—I was drowning again every time I was in a tight, enclosed space. The third was to understand and overcome the consequence of that belief. For me, it was a fear of travel, strong anxiety, and thoughts of mortality. In the end, I was able to turn around my thinking by learning to breathe in efficient ways designed to maximize my own oxygenation. By reinforcing in my mind that breathing (especially in tight spaces) was a positive experience—not a negative one—I was able to get back on solid ground.

It is impossible to overstate the power of oxygen in our lives. Oxygen heals. I've seen it in my professional practice and I practice what I teach in *my* everyday life. How many miraculous healing mechanisms can you name that are all around you at any given moment?

There's a reason renowned alternative therapy guru Gabriel Cousens calls oxygen "Vitamin O." He says, "Researchers have estimated that the amount of oxygen in the atmosphere two hundred years ago was 38 percent. Currently, it is 19 percent. In some cities, pollution is so severe that the amount of oxygen in the immediate atmosphere is as low as 12-14 percent."

Those figures leave little room for doubt that one of the major contributing factors to our current medical dilemmas is a basic lack of quality oxygen, and our collective neglect of its maintenance and consumption.

Every day, we're bombarded with health information ranging from diet tips to weight-loss secrets, even changing the flow of energy in your home and office. These tips are meant to highlight the cause of your problems, and how you can fix them in your quest for a healthy lifestyle. Yet, in the process of making these declarations, many self-proclaimed "experts" miss one of the most basic factors at the heart of a variety of ailments. Proper breathing is a factor that, when altered, can lead to balance and wellness throughout the body.

Think for a moment about how many breaths you take in your life. Start small: the average person takes about ten to twenty breaths in a single minute, which equals roughly 1,200 breaths in an hour, 28,800 per day. That's about ten million breaths in a single year! Obviously, breathing is an important function of the body's health and prosperity—it is life, after all. And yet, most people don't realize the true extent to which oxygen defines their quality of life.

While quality oxygen can help the body grow and thrive, it can also help repair damaged muscles and tissue from an injury or surgery. Brain cells die unless they receive proper oxygen. Yet most people are shallow breathers, and don't utilize the full spectrum of their breathing abilities. Put simply, while oxygen is freely available to use, most people do so inadequately; they don't use enough to help support full brain and body function.

New York Times wellness writer, Kris Carr, a cancer survivor, has a great analogy to explain what I mean: "If a fish is swimming in a dirty tank and it gets sick, do you take it to the vet and amputate the fin? No, you clean the water." In her quest for a better life after cancer, she cleaned up her system by eating organic raw greens and nuts, along with healthy fats. In doing so, she fueled her body with enzymes and vitamins, but also oxygen.

RECOVERING WITH OXYGEN THERAPY

As oxygenation has grown in popularity, rehabilitative therapies have emerged that incorporate the use of purified oxygen to help speed up the recovery process.

One of the most commonly used and well-known of these treatments is called Hyperbaric Oxygen Therapy (HBOT). HBOT dates back to the 17th century, but the modern medical community did not start studying it until after 1940.

You may remember the tabloids lambasting the pop singer Michael Jackson in the late '80s and early '90s, for reports that he slept every night in a hyperbaric chamber. For that supposed transgression, he was dubbed "Wacko Jacko" and shots of the singer inside his oxygen tent were highly coveted prizes in the paparazzi sweepstakes. What a difference education and further study has made in public perception.

Today, athletes like Tiger Woods use chambers installed in their homes to aid in injury recovery, and actor Keanu Reeves has used it to help with his insomnia. TV host Jenny McCarthy proclaimed on national television that she and her boyfriend at the time, actor Jim Carrey, each purchased hyperbaric chambers and even used them to help her son's autism. That was a major endorsement, one that brought to the mainstream a sensitive topic that nevertheless needs to be discussed: the potential benefits oxygen can have in the treatment of autism.

On the CBS's *The Doctors*, a show I'm proud to be a part of, professional football player Rodney Peete and his actress wife Holly Robinson Peete opened up about their struggles with an autistic son. Doctors told them their son would never compete athletically and never participate in mainstream schools—the prognosis was bleak. It was a touching episode that contained a surprising revelation: oxygen therapy helped their son improve his speech! Today, he's able to engage, has become quite vocal, and is "mainstreamed" in school. Rodney Peete eventually penned a book about his experience, titled *Not My Boy!*

With HBOT, patients enter a pressurized chamber that is saturated with quality oxygen. During the treatment, the oxygen is absorbed through the skin, and concentration in the tissues of any injury can increase up to twenty times at the cellular level. The treatment is painless and, most importantly, relaxing. Therapy can involve more than one treatment, and can last as long as necessary for the patient to feel fully recovered. Chambers include stand-up or bed-like units. Both types of systems deliver staggering results.

What makes HBOT so beneficial? First, HBOT facilitates cellular detoxification by creating an environment that is uninhabitable for bad bacteria, effectively cleansing the area and allowing productive bacterium to take the bad bacteria's place. HBOT can also greatly aid in the regeneration of nerves throughout the body. Nerves cannot survive without adequate supplies of clean, quality oxygen, and will actually regain use in the presence of the purified gas. HBOT can also help restore necessary oxygen stores to depleted tissues and cells that have been injured or impaired. Tissues and cells treated with oxygen therapy can actually return to full functioning levels after a period of time.

The American Cancer Society supports the use of HBOT, noting its proven effectiveness in recovery of over a dozen ailments, from embolisms to skin grafts and soft tissues. The University of California, which has an in-house HBOT chamber, lists some two-dozen problems it can help about 80 percent of the time.

The American Lung Association, which tends to be more restrictive with its backing of emerging science than other cancer organizations (the price that comes with being trusted by so many), states that oxygen therapy can improve patients' sleep and mood, as well as increase their mental alertness and stamina, allowing their bodies to carry out normal functions. It also prevents heart failure in people with severe lung disease.

The Mayo Clinic physician and research team includes board-certified specialists in undersea and hyperbaric medicine, who are also accredited by the Undersea and Hyperbaric Medical Society in conjunction with the Joint Commission. They are constantly looking for new and innovative ways to administer and perfect the use of oxygen therapy, and have one of the largest chambers in the country, capable of accommodating dozens of patients at once. How many oxygen treatments does the Mayo Clinic proudly claim it administers over the course of a single year? "Thousands," the organization's website boasts.

Hospitals all over the country are treating with oxygen therapy as well, including St. Joseph Hospital in Orange County, California; Abbott Northwestern in Minneapolis, Minnesota; William Beaumont Army Medical Center in El Paso, Texas; both Mount Sinai Hospital and New York Presbyterian in New York City. Soon, I expect HBOT will be a standard presence in most hospitals. In the often slow-moving field of medicine and emerging technology, the rush to be included in the next phase of successful treatment for a variety of ailments is an indication of what's to come.

In my own experience, I have seen impressive results with oxygen therapy. I once treated a patient who had experienced a lingual nerve injury in the third molar from anesthetics used during an extraction—a common occurrence that usually takes about six months to recover from. After eight sessions of HBOT over a course of roughly three months, the nerve was fully regenerated in half the time.

Some studies have shown that a series of HBOT sessions can improve healing by up to 30 percent, and that oxygen-supplementation treatments may be effective in patients suffering from a variety of different ailments. For example, in a test group of autistic children, 79 percent showed improvement in their levels of communication and motivation.

HBOT can also be highly effective for people with degenerative conditions. People who smoke or who are poor healers should seriously consider HBOT.

Conditions Helped with HBOT

- Alcoholism
- ADD/ADHD
- Arthritis
- Chronic fatigue syndrome
- Crohn's disease
- Decreased immune function, diabetes
- Fibromyalgia
- Learning disabilities
- Migraines
- Multiple Sclerosis
- Parkinson's disease
- Sports injuries
- Stroke
- Vascular disease

HBOT can also be used to prep patients for surgery, and help them recover after the operation. A health care provider can determine an adequate allotment of recovery time for a session of HBOT. While eight to ten sessions bring rapid and comprehensive recovery for many individuals, some heal more quickly and others need more sessions. Additionally, while full recovery may be experienced upon completion of the sessions, more time spent in the HBOT chamber can help resolve longstanding issues that existed prior to the injury or surgery. For instance, recent studies in cardiovascular literature suggest that patients undergoing open-heart surgery have better brain function if they receive treatment prior to their procedure. Other studies suggest oxygen treatment increases plasma concentration by ten to fifteen times, and that it can aid in reduction of swelling, inflammation, and promote growth of new blood vessels—an especially crucial benefit in facial reconstructions.

As it is with any medicine, there can be some complications associated with HBOT. During one study, in which more than seven hundred patients were followed for nearly twelve thousand therapy sessions, the most common complication was ear pain/discomfort in 17 percent of the patients. To minimize any risks of damage, techniques to clear the ears should be used during a session. Patients with hearing problems must take care to avoid damaging the hearing mechanism of the ears. While some participants in the study expressed concern about damage to lungs or teeth, no permanent damage of either was noted.

Although some long-term treatment options may be expensive, purchasing an HBOT chamber for the home can cost less than $5,000. However, since oxygen toxicity is a very rare side effect caused by getting too much oxygen too suddenly, your first session should be done in a professional setting, where prescreening is an important part of the process. Some companies lend and deliver chambers for home use on a weekly basis. Treatments range anywhere from $150 to $300 per session.

There's no magic pill that will help you heal faster than pressurized oxygen. And with today's consensus, there is simply no denying any longer the substantial benefits of oxygenation.

OZONE—A POWERFUL OXIDANT

In addition to HBOT, the use of ozonated treatments in medicinal or nutritional form has recently regained momentum among the general population.

For most people, the word "ozone" conjures up images of Earth's upper atmosphere. But ozone has many uses: bleaching, disinfecting the water supply, and keeping Jacuzzi water clean, to name a few. Water treatment research in Europe found that one molecule of ozone has the power of more than three thousand molecules of chlorine against different bacteria. The study demonstrated that ozone killed pathogenic or disease-causing organisms 3,500 times faster with no toxic side effects. Hundreds of medical ozone studies have demonstrated benefits such as improved wound healing and an accelerated immune system response.

Ozone was first described in the early 1800s. Nicola Tesla patented the first ozone generator in 1896. The Tesla Ozone Company was the first to administer ozone medically. Since then, ozone therapy has been used for a variety of issues. In the early 1900s, doctors published books and articles demonstrating the use of ozone in skin diseases and surgery. With the invention of antibiotics, ozone therapy fell out of favor, but because there is growing resistance to antibiotics because of the side effects due of overuse, ozone is making a big comeback. It's rising popularity is due in part to Ed McCabe, known in the industry as "Mr. Oxygen," who published a great book in 1988, *Oxygen Therapies, a New Way of Approaching Disease*. In it, he described all known oxygen therapies at the time that could eliminate disease and release toxins while activating the immune system.

Ozone also has the amazing ability to help the body stay free of disease-causing pathogens. It is a powerful oxidant against bacteria, viruses, fungi, and parasites. It destroys these invaders by burning holes through their cellular membranes, causing them to rupture. However, it is not harmful to human cells, due to the antioxidants present in the body.

In fact, ozone has a positive effect on cells: increasing their energy production. It enhances circulation by breaking up the clumping of the red blood cells at the site of an injury, allowing for better blood flow. It has a stimulatory effect on the immune system, increasing the number of white blood cells in the tissues. Treatment can be used intravenously or can be injected at the site of injury to help reduce excessive inflammation and pain and accelerate healing.

Frank Shallenberger, MD, considered a leader in ozone therapy, treats a variety of degenerative, chronic, and autoimmune diseases. He reports that ozone has the ability to stop tumor progression.

In 1983, the World Ozone Conference officially announced that ozone can successfully treat HIV, herpes, liver problems including cirrhosis, non-healing ulcers, cardiovascular disease, tumors, cancers, arthritis, allergies, yeast infections, and parasites. Ozone can also be applied on the skin's surface to help with wound healing, including postsurgical wounds and open sores.

When administered properly as a treatment for healing, ozone is safe. The two human tissues that can be irritated by ozone are the lungs and the eyes. So while a small amount in the atmosphere is tolerable, pure ozone is never used in medicine. It is always mixed with oxygen. In the medical office, ozone gas is used at a concentration of 0.05 percent to maximum 5 percent in the ozone to oxygen ratio. To make ozone in the office, oxygen is passed through an ozone generator at different concentrations depending on the need. A lower concentration is typically used when directly injected under the skin, into the blood, or into a muscle.

Ozone treatment is used in the dental field. Since the purified oxygen mixed with the ozone eradicates the bad bacteria in a specific area, it can be used eliminate these intruders in small cracks within teeth and in other hard-to-reach oral canals and fissures.

In my practice, I use ozone routinely, in the form of gas or ozonated water, to treat dental hypersensitivity and oral ulcers. I also use ozone to:

- Disinfect the mouth as a pre-treatment rinse before surgery

- Keep the water supply bottles of the hand pieces bacteria-free

- Treat gingival inflammation and reverse cavities

- Treat abscesses—we use low-concentration ozone injections in lieu of antibiotics

- Disinfect the office air from the aerosols caused by the dental drill

Since ozone is composed of molecules that are stable only for short periods of time—typically one to two days—ozonated water cannot be effectively bottled. However, there are some home units to generate ozonated water for daily rinsing. The home units are not as strong as professional ones, but they may suffice for someone suffering from mouth sores.

In an effort to shed light on the health science behind oxygen and ozone therapy, the Department of Psychology at Vanderbilt University recently tackled the subject and arrived at some mind-blowing results. Its report, titled "The Real Story Behind Oxygen Therapy," states that: "Ozone therapy, like oxidative therapy, is very effective because rather than intoxicating the liver and other organs with drugs, ozone therapy involves oxidizing 'the molecules in the shell of the virus." The report explains how during treatment, the ozone molecules "give up their third oxygen atom, releasing considerable energy which destroys all lipid-enveloped viruses, and apparently all other disease organisms, while leaving the blood cells unharmed. Moreover, the blood becomes oxygenated more sufficiently than it normally does, although this may seem hard to believe considering the fact that hemoglobin is so efficient." The treatment involves withdrawing blood, infusing it with oxygen, and then injecting it back into the patient, at which point the report elaborates on how "the strengthened blood confers some of its virucidal properties to the rest of the patient's blood as it disperses, finally evening out in the end to reach equilibrium. The patient's state then remains the same provided he exercises, diets, and breathes deeply regularly."

The American Cancer Society stops short of fully backing ozone therapy, but it does note: "Ozone and hydrogen peroxide are known to have properties of disinfection, much like chlorine bleach, and are often used to clean instruments or surfaces. They are used in careful concentrations to clean or disinfect wounds ... There are differences in the way cancer cells use oxygen that may allow new treatments to better target cancer cells."

OZONATED OILS—LONGER LASTING

Ozonated options have now expanded to include oils, including olive, jojoba, sesame seed, coconut, and peanut. Ozonated oils are much more effective at delivering topical ozone than ozonated water; water can only hold the added oxygen for a short period of time, while ozonated oils can last several months on the shelf.

Ozonated oils are known for their antibacterial and healing properties, and can be used on a variety of ailments for immediate and long-term results, without side effects. For instance, an estimated one and a half billion people suffer from skin-related conditions—a number that is expected to rise along with the increasing rates of inflammation and obesity. Topical antibacterial and corticosteroid medication to remedy skin ailments can be expensive enough without having to also medicate the side effects that occur. Furthermore, antibacterial and corticosteroid medications can slow down healing. And while micro-organisms are starting to be resistant to topical antibiotics, no resistance to ozone has been found.

A study presented in 2011, in the journal *Mycoses*, looked at four hundred patients suffering from a fungal infection of the skin. Half of the group was treated with ozonated sunflower oil (Oleozon) and the other half with an antifungal cream. Oleozon was 90 percent effective in getting rid of the infection, while the antifungal was only 13 percent effective.

Ozonated oils can be applied topically for cuts, scrapes, wounds, and for bacterial or fungal infections. Oxygen is absorbed through the skin and enters the circulatory system, so it not only has a local effect but a systemic effect, even when applied on the surface of the skin. Topical application of ozonated oils speeds up the healing process by going deep within the wound to bring blood flow to the area and decrease pain.

Ozonated oil can also be consumed orally for positive effects inside the body. It can be used to treat conditions in the mouth, such as canker sores and ulcers, without the side effects associated with many medications. If several are present, a tablespoon of ozonated oil can be swished around inside the mouth for as long as possible, and then swallowed. The treatment should be repeated four times a day, until the areas heal.

The process of making these oils is lengthy and must be done properly in order to be effective. For instance, when making ozonated olive oil, ozone gas is bubbled inside oil typically for a couple of weeks to create the final product. Since quality is so important, it is best to purchase ozonated oils from a reputable company.

Compared to other options, whether topical or systemic, such as the hyperbaric chamber, ozonated oils are relatively inexpensive and very effective, without side effects. They are definitely worth a try!

DEEP BREATHING—HEAL WITH THE AIR AROUND YOU

Ultimately, while there are many factors to consider when looking at overall healing, oxygen, as you've read, is absolutely one of the most important.

In the quest for accelerated recovery, remembering to intake large quantities of quality oxygen is one of the easiest ways to move forward on the path to a healthy and happy lifestyle.

In his book, *The Oxygen Breakthrough,* Sheldon Hendler, PhD, described how deep breathing can positively influence all aspects of health, and how, with deep breathing, his patients were able to get off the majority of their medications. Best of all, it's free—so don't underestimate the power of deep breathing.

It can be difficult to alter a lifelong habit of shallow breathing, but the good news is that you can change your oxygen levels with breathing exercises.

The Alexander Technique is a great way to retrain the chest and stomach muscles that control breathing. The technique helps you learn how to release tension, breathe deeply, and connect to your breath. Developed in the 1940s, the Alexander Technique can also help relieve pain from repetitive strain injury, backache, stiff neck, and shoulders. A study in 2008, published in the *British Medical Journal*, confirmed the effectiveness of the Alexander Technique in treating back pain. I highly advise you to seek out a trained practitioner in your area to help you get started. The Alexander Technique is part of a general field of practice known as "breath work," which has the goal of increasing your oxygen levels through conscious breathing from the diaphragm.

When stressed, a person tends to breathe from the chest because the muscles tense and don't allow the movement of the ribs or stomach. In normal deep breathing, the breath should go all the way to the stomach; you should see the rise and fall of your belly button with every inhale and exhale. Take a deep breath now, and expand your stomach as far as it'll go.

MEASURING OXYGEN LEVELS AT OUR CLINIC

Oxygen level in the tissues is measured with a pulse oximeter, a device placed on a finger that reads the percentage of oxygen saturation in an instant. Nail polish must be removed to get an accurate reading with the device. A pulse oximeter is commonly used by health professionals, including dentists, as a tool for monitoring vital signs. Oxygen saturation should typically measure around 99 percent. If your oxygen saturation is lower than that, your tissues are not getting the oxygen they need. Poor breathing can result in muscle cramps, high blood pressure, hormonal imbalances, and chronic fatigue.

When practicing deep breathing or breath work, inhale through the nose, not through the mouth. The nostrils filter air, acting as a purifier before are reaches the lungs. Mouth breathing long-term can create numerous problems, including dry mouth and red and swollen gums in the front of the mouth. These conditions are difficult to treat unless mouth breathing stops. In children, mouth breathing can even cause skeletal problems, including alterations of the facial structure. By practicing simple daily deep breathing techniques through the nose, mouth breathing can be stopped.

I was fortunate to participate in a ninety-minute session of deep breathing guided by a therapist at a retreat in Palm Springs a few years ago. The seminar, titled "Breath Work," involved breathing to consciously connect oxygen throughout the body. It was an amazing experience and I highly recommend it. The breath work included some of my favorite—and some of the most regenerative—breathing exercises, such as the "Lion's Breath" and "Breath of Fire."

I recommend doing breathing exercises on a daily basis, for at least five minutes. This can be incorporated as part of your meditation, or just as a quick exercise on its own. A number of audio files and apps are available online to help you get started learning to breath deeply.

Here's a simple breathing exercise that I recommend doing every day. When starting out, try to do a minimum of five minutes.

- Sit in a comfortable position with your back straight and arms by your side.

- Inhale through the nose, slowly counting to four, and feel your stomach expanding.

- Hold the breath for a count of two or longer, depending on your comfort.

- Exhale through the nose slowly on a count of four.

- Hold for a count of two or longer before inhaling again.

Notice how great you will feel from doing the simple exercise. As you practice deep breathing, you will feel new levels of energy and the sense of calmness. It will also improve your sleep.

Let me say it again: oxygen heals. I've watched it help patients in my professional practice and I've experienced its healing power myself.

The quality of the oxygen you take in also shouldn't be taken for granted. Perhaps no other story serves as a better than a patient of mine who had overcome lung cancer. When I asked him how he was able to overcome it, I assumed he had undergone treatment.

"Was it chemotherapy? Surgery?" I asked.

"No," he replied. "I have done neither of those."

Turns out, he went to a retreat in northern California where he was surrounded by loved ones, ate clean food, and, perhaps most importantly, breathed clean air. When he went back to the oncologist eight months later, he was completely free and clear of cancer.

University studies confirm the benefits of oxygen, and major health organizations have had to admit that oxygen—in whatever ways it's distributed to patients—improves overall health.

As I mentioned at the beginning of this chapter, "experts" will look to anything other than the fundamental basics and the building blocks of the entire world to find solutions. I've always maintained that this hyper-targeting of specific areas—weight loss, heart-healthy diets, trendy exercise routines—completely misses the point of general, overall health. The key is to reconnect with your environment, and there's nothing more all-encompassing than the air we breathe.

Use it wisely, use it liberally. Inhale the benefits. Start right now! Take a deep breath and, just like that, you're on the right path to a healthier you.

....

CHAPTER 6

HEALING WITH PLANTS, HERBS, AND TEAS

Today, nearly one-third of Americans are using herbs, and the World Health Organization estimates that 80 percent of people in the world use herbal remedies.

Herbs are not a recent evolution of medicine or a new trend in what people subscribe to. Using herbs is more of a movement in which people are remembering what has worked for thousands of years.

I have a long history with herbal remedies, stretching all the way back to my childhood in Romania. I have fond memories of going through the forest near my home and harvesting plants for teas. My grandmother used to sun-dry all kinds of medicinal plants, flowers, and seeds, then store them in jars for different ailments.

Plants have been used for medicinal purposes long before recorded history. There are writings from the ancient Chinese and Egyptian cultures recording the medical uses for plants dating as far back as early 3,000 BC. Perhaps what is most interesting is that different cultures in different parts of the world have historically devised the same medicinal uses for certain plants, using the same parts of the plants in the same amounts.

Plants and herbs are no secret to the pharmaceutical industry. In fact, medicines often try to mimic and magnify the healing attributes of different extracts of plants and herbs. However, in isolating the different components of the herb and magnifying them well beyond their natural purpose, the work of pharmaceutical companies then becomes *un*natural and can do more harm than good. The result is often unwanted side effects.

The following is a quick glimpse into some of the must-haves that I keep in my medicine cabinet and recommend to my patients for healing. These represent just a brief sampling of the many healing plants out there. I encourage you to do additional research or consult with an herbalist on other resources that may be best for your specific concerns.

HEALING THROUGH ESSENTIAL OILS

I have been using essential oils in my life and in my practice for several years. It's a therapy modality that I recommend for everyday use. Most essential oils are known for their antibacterial qualities, as well as a wide spectrum of other health benefits. Some of those benefits include anti-inflammatory, antiviral, anti-parasitic, anti-fungal, anti-septic, sedative, regenerating, uplifting, restorative, oxygenating, and analgesic. Essential oils can help accelerate healing by giving your body some of the nutrients it needs at that particular time. That, in turn, helps facilitate a faster and more comfortable recovery period.

I recommend using certified pure therapeutic-grade essential oils whenever possible. Other oils may smell just as good, but they will be missing a lot of the ingredients that are beneficial to healing, and ultimately may not produce the desired effect. Certified, pure oils are a perfect distillation of the plant, and have a higher concentration of the physical properties of the flowers and plants from which they are derived. For that reason, a little bit goes a long way.

Essential oils can be administered orally, inhaled, or applied topically; either neat (with no dilution), or via compresses or baths. Let me briefly explain the guidelines for each of these uses.

Ingesting Essential Oils. Remember that essential oils are already a very concentrated form of the plant they've come from. When taking internally, it's best to consult with an experienced, qualified health expert to ensure the oil is a good oral remedy for the condition you want to treat. The FDA has approved some essential oils for oral administration, and these have been given the label GRAS (Generally Recognized As Safe). Before ingesting any oil, make sure it has the GRAS classification.

Generally, an oral dose will impact your internal environment eight to ten times more than any other form of administration. Although that might sound favorable, more doesn't necessarily mean better results. It's easier to overdose on an oil when it is used incorrectly, and the dangers vary from oil to oil. Rosemary oil, for example, is recognized as safe by the FDA, but should be avoided by patients with high blood pressure and by pregnant women. That's why it's best to get clear guidelines on how much you should be taking internally of any essential oil you're not familiar with.

The flip side is that ingesting them can be a faster way to get the healing components into your system. When used correctly, ingesting oil is a powerful agent to accelerate your recovery.

Essential oils can be incorporated into everyday cooking. Just remember that one drop of certified grade therapeutic oil may be enough, since it is so concentrated. One of my favorites is vanilla-lavender frozen yogurt. You can also use the healing lemon oil to make salad dressings. In the summertime, I like to flavor my drinking water with grapefruit or mint essential oil.

GRAS CLASSIFIED ESSENTIAL OILS

Angelica	Grapefruit	Peppermint
Basil	Hyssop	Petitgrain
Bergamot	Juniper	Pine
Chamomile,	Jasmine	Rosemary
Roman	Laurus nobilis	Rose
Chamomile,	Lavender	Savory
German	Lemon	Sage
Cinnamon bark	Lemongrass	Sandalwood
Clary sage	Lime	Spearmint
Clove	Melissa	Spruce
Coriander	Marjoram	Tarragon
Eucalyptus globulus	Myrrh	Tangerine
Frankincense	Myrtle	Thyme
Galbanum	Nutmeg	Valerian
Geranium	Orange	Vertiver
Ginger	Oregano	Ylang Ylang

Inhaling Essential Oils. Scents can have a powerful effect on the body. Just consider the last time you walked past a freshly cut lawn and the memories that flooded back to you. Perhaps there's a certain cologne or perfume that has you reminiscing of a lost love. A whiff of certain spices might put you back in your grandmother's kitchen in an instant.

We've all had these experiences and they are real. Your sense of smell is tied into your limbic system, which is made up of the parts of your brain that deal with things like your emotions, behaviors, motivations, and long-term memory. When you inhale different essential oils, they can trigger your brain to release certain chemicals into the body that calm you and create a real, measurable, physical experience. That experience can release stress, helping to ease the burden on your body and creating an environment in which your immune system can thrive.

You can inhale these oils by holding an open bottle of pure oil up to your nose. Or, by using a cold diffuser, you can distribute the oils into the air, allowing you to regularly breathe them in. The oil molecules remain suspended in the air for several hours. The amount of oil available to inhale is greatly reduced over holding the bottle of oil to your nose because it is much more diluted by being dispersed into the air. However, that is somewhat offset by the amount of time you are exposed to the oil, as you can you leave the diffuser on for long periods of time and experience the rejuvenating effects of the scent whenever you are in the room throughout your day. The cold diffusion of oils kills bacteria and mold, and also reduces the chemical load of the air you breathe.

You can expect to experience lifted moods, greater energy, and a sense of calm and relaxation—depending on the oils used. Relaxation accelerates healing just like stress discourages it. That's why I recommend essential oils during recovery. One of my very favorite oils to use is lavender, both for its calming effect and the list of other health benefits it offers.

I love to put a couple of drops of oil in the shower for a quick way to perk up in the morning. If you don't have a diffuser, you can also use a cup with hot water; just add a couple of drops of oil and inhale. Frankincense oil, when inhaled, powers up the immune system by increasing the activity of the white blood cells to fight against infections. It also has powerful anti-inflammatory properties.

Topical Application of Essential Oils. Essential oils can be applied topically to the skin and problem areas of the body. Certain oils can even be applied on an open wound to help stop bleeding and promote disinfection. Helichrysum and clove oil can be applied to an open wound, one drop each, to help stop bleeding and decrease the pain.

Clove oil is one of my favorites in my practice. Due to its analgesic effect, it's a great topical pain relief for after gingival grafting, or any oral wound. It can be added to fractionated coconut oil (fractionated oils are refined to remove some components) for dilution, and used for a toothache for immediate relief.

In dentistry, eugenol has been extracted from clove and incorporated as part of a zinc oxide dental paste to be used in root canal treatments. If a patient develops a dry socket following a wisdom tooth extraction, a eugenol paste is applied directly to the site and left overnight to calm the area and promote healing and disinfection. Historically, clove has also been used for skin infections in medicine and for bad breath, due to its anti-infectious and anti-bacterial properties.

Lavender oil works great to relax the muscles. It has an immediate calming effect. Eucalyptus oil also works the same way. When applied topically, these oils should be diluted into something else, such as a lotion or another oil, known as a carrier oil. Personally, I prefer to use coconut oil, which is beneficial for better cells, nerves, and hormonal health. There's no exact science to how many drops of the essential oil to use, but a good rule of thumb is to use about eight to ten drops per two teaspoons of carrier oil, which is equal to about twenty drops per one ounce.

Once the oils are mixed, simply rub the concoction on the areas where you want relief. The skin has an amazing capacity to absorb nutrients. The areas of the body that absorb oils the fastest are the feet (due to the large amount of pores), behind the ears, and on the wrists. A 1992 study showed that two of the chemicals in lavender, linalool, and linalyl acetate, were absorbed through the abdominal skin and carried into the blood plasma within minutes.

Applying essential oils to reflexology points in the hands and feet, is a great way to administer treatment. Via these points, the oil can have a therapeutic effect on the internal organs. A reflexology chart is included later in the chapter.

Compresses using essential oils are very useful and effective when either hot or cold. Following oral surgery, for example, cold compresses can be used to decrease inflammation. Add a few drops of oil to cold water then soak a towel fully. Rinse out the excess water and place the compress over the inflamed area of the face. The compress can also be applied to other parts of the body, but not directly to an open wound.

I use essential oils in my practice as well. For instance, I'm often working with patients who have pain that comes from TMJ, or grinding or clenching their teeth at night. For them, I massage the oil into the jaw area, allowing it to penetrate deep into the joint and muscle. The result is that the inflammation diminishes and they are able to find relief from pain.

Due to the antibacterial properties of essential oils, I recommend some of them to be used to treat inflammation in the mouth. A drop of Thieves (a powerful combination) oil or melaleuca (tea tree) oil can be added to toothpaste to treat gingivitis. Today, many toothpaste brands already contain essential oils, with melaleuca being a popular one. I don't recommend using melaleuca oil on a regular basis to brush your teeth, because it is too strong and it also kills off beneficial bacteria. You may experience actual sloughing (shedding skin) of the gums since it is such a strong oil to be used every day.

Don't forget about using essential oils in the bath! But be careful not to add too much, as they can irritate the skin. Three to six drops is the recommended dose to be added to running water. The oil particles will disperse and they can be easily absorbed through the skin.

CHOOSING THE RIGHT KIND OF OILS

Essential oils are *not* the same thing as fragrance oils. Essential oils are derived from plants, while fragrance oils are manufactured in labs. The latter are artificially engineered, and often include synthetic chemicals that are harmful to your body. Although fragrances smell good, that is their only benefit.

However, even when buying the real deal—true essential oils—take care with your selections. The purest oils will always come from cold extractions. For further guidance, consider consulting a qualified professional about what is considered a reputable brand. Generally, look for therapeutic grade oils, not just plain essential oils.

The following charts do not include all essential oils available. It is provided to give guidance for someone who is beginning to use essential oils for their own personal use.

Antibacterial	Antifungal	Antiparasitic	Antiviral
Basil	Clove	Clove	Clove
Clove	Geranium	Oregano	Eucalyptus
Geranium	Tea tree		Tea tree
Grapefruit	Oregano		Myrrh
Lemon	Thyme		
Orange			
Oregano			
Tea tree			

Anti-inflammatory	Pain control	Immune system	Antidepressant
Basil	Eucalyptus	Frankincense	Frankincense
Bergamot	Ginger	Lemon	Geranium
Chamomile	Lavender	Oregano	Lavender
Lavender	Lemongrass	Rosemary	Orange
Lemongrass	Oregano	Thyme	Sandalwood
Myrrh	Peppermint	Tea tree	
Peppermint			

Antioxidant	Bruises	Fatigue	Swelling
Clove	Geranium	Peppermint	Cypress
Thyme	Helichrysum	Basil	Grapefruit
Rosemary	Fennel	Lemongrass	Lemongrass
Peppermint			

EMERGENCY ESSENTIAL OILS

Essential oils can have anywhere from two hundred to eight hundred active ingredients, and it's believed that there may even be many more in some oils.

I recommend keeping certain oils on hand in case of an emergency; however, due to the plethora of active ingredients, you only need a handful of them to cover different problems:

- Clove oil is great for pain relief. It is also a great antiseptic. It can be applied in the mouth and on the body.

- Lavender can be used topically for bruises, burns, insect bites, and sunburn. It is also good for anxiety when diffused in the room.

- Frankincense facilitates recovery from any surgery or injury and helps with fatigue.

- Oregano can be used as an antibiotic went ingested. When placed on the bottoms of the feet, it can actually be tasted in the mouth.

- Peppermint is a great topical pain relief and can also be used for fever and nausea.

- Tea tree (melaleuca) oil can be used inside the mouth to relieve gum inflammation and sore throat. It can also be used on the skin for inflammation such as eczema or wounds.

TEAS AND HERBAL SUPPLEMENTS

Another way to benefit from the medicinal value of plants is to take them in tea form. Looking back in the history of natural medicine, healing teas were used over five thousand years ago, and medicinal plants even earlier than that. Ancient healers and physicians used to mix their own herbal teas and prescribed them for different ailments. Many of these recipes have been passed down from generation to generation. Modern pharmacology uses some of these extracts for drug formulations today. In the United States, people are rediscovering the therapeutic effects of teas, and the consumption of teas increases by 8 to 10 percent every year.

I have a real connection to teas as a source of healing because they were such a personal part of my life growing up in Romania. We grew up very close to a mountainous area, and you could often find

PREPARING TEA

Here are some general rules for getting the most out of the plant when preparing tea:

- Use filtered water. Tap water can contain many chemicals that may interfere with the properties of the tea.

- Only use stainless steel, glass, or porcelain for steeping tea. Do not use aluminum or plastic containers, which can alter the taste of the tea.

- Follow the instructions for steeping a particular tea. Overboiling may destroy valuable properties of the brew.

- Do not add sweetener. If sweetener is a must-have, use a bit of raw honey or xylitol.

- If using fresh herbs, you will need roughly twice as much plant as using dried herbs.

my family walking through the forest, picking different plants for their medicinal value and breathing in the fresh air. Today, there is still nothing quite like a cup of freshly harvested Romanian Elderflower tea.

Teas are great to recuperate during healing. They help to hydrate and contain phytochemicals, which can act like antioxidants to provide a wide variety of benefits that support healing before, during, and after bouts of illness or physical trauma.

THE ROLE OF ANTIOXIDANTS

It is especially important to ensure the proper intake of antioxidants during periods of sickness and healing; that is when the body creates more free radicals than any other period of time. Think of inflammation as the fire and antioxidants as being the water to put out the fire. To put out the fire, the body needs two to three times more antioxidants when it is inflamed and needing to heal. When your body is in a weakened state, it is more susceptible to viruses and bacteria, which means you are more likely to get sick. Since everything in the body is interconnected—one system affects another—even an injury that is technically confined to one area of the body puts stress on the whole body.

Teas for Antioxidants. Your body requires antioxidants to be able to fight against free radicals (covered in chapter 1), which can cause the DNA inside the cells to mutate. That activity can result in different diseases and potentially cause cancer, if the body doesn't have the ability to repair the damage. But as desperately as your body needs antioxidants, it is not able to produce any on its own. That means it is entirely dependent on what it takes in from nature, which means it is entirely dependent on *you*.

Teas are a very effective way to take in a lot of antioxidants at once, and green tea is one that is very well known for its antioxidant and anti-inflammatory properties. There are records of green tea being used in China five thousand years ago. Today, more people drink green tea than any other beverage outside of water. A considerable amount of research in recent years has shown how effective green tea is in repairing DNA damage, lowering incidence of heart disease and stroke, and reducing the risk of cancer. Green tea has been shown to fight dental decay and bad breath, although it's not a substitute for brushing and flossing.

Green tea is rich in polyphenols, potent antioxidants that help fight oxidative stress from everyday life or during healing; excessive stress causes more free radicals to be released, disrupting cellular membranes and potentially causing disease. EGCG (epigallocatechin gallate), one of the polyphenols found in green tea, has been shown to be a stronger antioxidant than vitamins E or C. People who drink green tea daily have a much lower incidence of tumors found in the liver, skin, lungs, and esophagus. Red, black, and white teas are also very high in antioxidants.

Teas for Accelerated Healing and Immunity. Different teas have various health benefits that can assist in speedy recovery, and help strengthen the body against disease. Teas also contain a variety of minerals, which are beneficial for a healthy immune system. Like antioxidants, teas that strengthen the immune system, or have antiviral and antibacterial properties, can help prevent the onset of sickness. For example, horsetail contains calcium, copper, selenium, and zinc. Horsetail is a medicinal plant that is known to treat fractured bones and connective tissues.

Elderberry tea, which is also high in antioxidants, is often used as an herbal supplement to strengthen the immune system. Taking an immune booster, like elderberry or Echinacea, can help strengthen your immune system and protect you from disease. These are also helpful for people who are already sick or who have undergone any kind of physical trauma, such as surgery or an injury.

Elderberry can also be administered in syrup form. When patients come in with colds, coughs, or similar ailments, I am quick to recommend a trip to the store to pick up some elderberry extract.

TEAS TO ACCELERATE HEALING

I strongly recommend teas with high antiviral and antibacterial properties to help accelerate your healing, and protect you during recovery. The two that I use most often are goldenseal and Echinacea. These have such high properties that I use them as an adjunct to antibiotics in my practice.

Ginger tea from fresh ginger is also known as an antibacterial against colds and flu, but it is also popularly known for its ability to help a person overcome nausea from antibiotics or IV sedation. Ginger increases circulation, directing more nutrients to the site and enhancing the immune function to facilitate healing.

Although I am not advocating using herbs in place of antibiotics (especially postoperatively or for acute infection), in some cases, herbs can play a key role in the treatment of low-grade chronic conditions. Some of these include: goldenseal, calendula, and licorice. Licorice is also anti-inflammatory and I like to use it whenever an anti-inflammatory medication is recommended.

It is best to consult your health specialist before taking any herbs to ensure you are using the right dosage. Some of them may interact with medications you are already taking, and some can actually be toxic if taken in high quantities. Just because it is natural, doesn't mean it is safe.

When your body is healing, it's also very important to get proper rest and relaxation. But it can be difficult to get proper rest and relaxation if your body is in constant pain, because dealing with that pain can raise your stress levels and make it difficult to get comfortable. Teas can be used to help facilitate a more comfortable and relaxed physical state.

My absolute favorite tea comes from the elderflower, which I picked all my life in Romania. It comes from the same tree as the elderberry, which has the loveliest fragrance. The flower is a nervine, meaning it helps to calm the nervous system. Linden tea is a wonderful nighttime tea as well. I always have a selection of teas on hand, as enjoying tea is a regular part of my life. Other popular nervines include valerian, lavender, and chamomile.

If you are not a fan of tea, the benefits of these herbs can be obtained in capsule or tincture form.

CHOOSING THE RIGHT HERBS

It's impossible to be too picky when it comes to selecting the right distributor for your herbal teas and supplements. The FDA regulates the herbal industry. Yet, the shelves are lined with dead herbs that have no medicinal value at all—despite promises on the bottle. Don't believe everything you read.

The best way to ensure you are getting the quality you deserve is to consult with a qualified professional—a doctor, nutritionist, acupuncturist, or other trusted source—that is familiar with proven, high-quality distributors. It can be difficult to decipher the research and published viability presented by the different companies out there, but a qualified professional will be able to crack the code and give you sound guidance on "who's who" in the industry.

One of the best tips I can offer you is to always stick with organic or wild-crafted herbs. Otherwise, you risk ingesting a product that is riddled with chemicals and pesticides. Some companies even bleach their herbs as part of the process. Of course, you can always go the very traditional route and select your own wild-crafted herbs. That means they are freshly harvested, which eliminates a lot of steps between getting it from the ground to the body. Fresh harvesting is a great way to preserve a lot of the vitality of the plant for your benefit.

I have the most affinity to wild-crafted herbs. To this day, my mom always gathers a fresh harvest of elderflower during her trips back to Romania. When she comes home, we sit and talk about her trip over a nice, hot cup of tea.

Here are some herbs that are ideal for boosting the immune system. Below, I've listed herbs that help to soothe and calm you.

Immune Boosting Herbs

Astragalus is one of the most famous Chinese tonic herbs and is often used to boost the immune system. It can be found in tablet form for can be made into a tea.

Bee pollen has been used for centuries as a superfood. It has antibiotic, antiviral, and antifungal properties. It is a powerhouse of vitamins and minerals. It's great for taking during recovery.

Echinacea is a plant that has been used for thousands of years by Native Americans for infections and wounds. It is a powerful immune-system stimulant that is also available as a tincture or tablets. It is oftentimes found in combination with goldenseal. Echinacea root in a mouthwash can be used to alleviate mouth ulcers.

Garlic is an antiseptic with antibiotic, antiparasitic, and anti-fungal action. Its active ingredient, allicin, also aids circulatory problems by lowering blood pressure and reducing cholesterol. Garlic can be used to treat infections of the mouth, throat, and digestive tract.

Ginkgo biloba can be used as a tea, tincture, or tablets to improve circulation, blood flow, and oxygenation. It also has antioxidant and anti-inflammatory properties.

Ginseng has been used to strengthen the immune system for thousands of years. It is also used as a tonic in stress and after prolonged illness. It is available as a tea, tincture, or tablets.

Goldenseal can be used as an antiseptic remedy for inflammation, sore throats, mouth sores, gum disease, and digestive problems. It has a reputation of "cure-all," because it is good for any infection for the whole body.

Milk thistle strengthens and clears the liver and gallbladder, especially for those taking several medications. It is also useful for inflammation caused by candida (gut yeast) infection. Tell your doctor if you're planning to take this in conjunction with other medications.

Pau d'arco is a super-powerful tea that comes from the bark of a tree native to Brazil. It has antibacterial, antiviral, antiparasitic, anticancer, and anti-inflammatory properties that have been confirmed scientifically. It is used to treat ulcers, allergies, infections, and many other diseases. The tea must be boiled for ten to fifteen minutes to extract all the active ingredients.

Sage has a mild anti-inflammatory effect, and can be used as a spray or tea to improve sore throat, canker sores, and gingivitis. It also helps with intestinal cramping and improves the memory.

Calming and Soothing Herbs

Aloe Vera is a tropical plant that is commonly used for cuts, scrapes, and burns. Fresh aloe vera is best, as many of the enzymes are alive. The gel inside the plant is soothing and cooling and has antibacterial and antifungal functions. The plant can be easily grown in a small pot either inside or outside. Studies have shown that it shortens healing time of cuts and wounds, as well as herpes outbreaks. I recommend this to my patients for any ulceration or inflammation inside the mouth, either in the form of a juice for fresh plant. The aloe vera should have contact with the affected area for as long as possible.

Calendula or marigold flowers have been recommended for a variety of inflammatory skin conditions such as eczema. The flavonoids in the yellow pigment of the plant gives it its anti-inflammatory quality. It can be applied topically to the affected area in the form of a cream or gel. It can also be used as a tea, tincture, or compress.

Chamomile is a calming agent great for headaches, stress, and insomnia. It helps with digestive cramps and can be taken as a tea or tincture. Long-term use offers better results.

Comfrey can be used as a topical tincture, compress, or lotion to relieve pain and to speed up healing of cuts, bruises, broken bones, and wounds. Comfrey is also good as a cream for dry and cracked skin. It should not be used internally because it has been shown to cause liver disease in rats.

Kombucha has become a widely popular tea. It is fermented green tea made from a mushroom, and contains beneficial probiotics.

Although no in-depth studies have been done, it is reported that it may strengthen the immune system, increase energy levels, and detoxify the digestive tract.

Mushroom tea, made of medicinal mushrooms such as reishi, shiitake, chaga, and cordyceps, can be brewed to make a potent immuno-stimulant. I'll discuss medicinal mushrooms in-depth in the next chapter.

Parsley, in addition to being a tasty condiment, can also be made into tea for use against fluid retention and swelling. The roots are more powerful than the leaves.

St. John's wort, used as a tea or tincture, is useful for nerve pain and relaxation. It strengthens and speeds the healing of the nervous system. It is a good alternative to prescription medication for pain, and should not be taken in conjunction with pain medications as it may interact.

Valerian is available as a tea or tincture, and can be used as a natural sedative in place of sleeping medications. Valerian is not physically addictive, unlike benzodiazepines, but people can become dependent on it. Do not mix it with any antidepressants.

Condition	Medicinal herbs
Allergies	Echinacea, garlic, licorice, pau d'arco
Bone injuries	Comfrey (external), dandelion, horsetail
Burns	Calendula, comfrey
Circulation	Garlic, ginkgo, ginger, licorice
Edema (swelling)	Parsley
Fever	Calendula, chamomile, feverfew
Immunity	Astragalus, echinacea, garlic, ginseng, goldenseal, pau d'arco
Infection	Echinacea, garlic, goldenseal, licorice, pau d'arco

Condition	Medicinal herbs
Insomnia	Chamomile, St. John's wort, velarium
Nausea	Anise, ginger, peppermint
Oral problems	Goldenseal, green tea, sage
Pain	Capsicum, chamomile, comfrey, valerian
Wounds	Comfrey (external), goldenseal, peppermint, horsetail

The medicinal herbs I mentioned in this chapter are just a select few that are easily found over-the-counter to alleviate pain and accelerate healing. They are by no means a complete list or an alternative to seeking medical advice.

CHAPTER 7

....

HEALING WITH VITAMINS AND SUPPLEMENTS

S hortly after Chelsea had a dental implant placed, it failed. It simply did not integrate and finally loosened. Chelsea was a vegan and had many gaps in her daily diet and nutritional needs. Coincidentally, she also had patches of skin irritation around her scalp and elbows. She reported going to the dermatologist, who thought she had psoriasis, but no medicated cream relieved her symptoms. She was more frustrated with the skin irritation than she was with the failed implant.

After a personalized consultation, I had her start taking a multi-vitamin/mineral formulation to promote healing of bone and skin. The dental implant was reworked and three months later, it was healing fine. Remarkably, her skin irritation was also healing and nearly disappeared.

Inflammation, as you'll recall from the introduction, is the body's first response following an injury, whether from a sports activity, surgery, or an invasion of bacteria or a virus. It is the stage in the healing process that promotes the gathering of cells to the injured organ, tissues, bones, or joint, in order to start the repair process. If the inflammation does not subside after a few days and continues for more than a week, then the inflammation is considered to be chronic.

Although "Inflammation is not a disease," according to Howard Loomis Jr., DC, FIACA, author of the book *Enzymes: The Key to Health, Volume I*, today, inflammation is treated like a disease that must be suppressed with anti-inflammatory medications.

The most frequently prescribed medications worldwide are non-steroidal anti-inflammatory drugs, also known as NSAIDs. In the United States alone, over seventy million prescriptions for NSAIDs are written every year, and millions more are sold over-the-counter. Many people take these drugs like candy, without thinking twice of their side effects. In 2015, the European Union cautioned against NSAIDs due to their association with a higher increase in cardiovascular problems, heart attacks, and strokes. Other side effects include gastrointestinal bleeding, kidney failure, liver toxicity, and dizziness. People who use NSAIDs are four times more likely to be hospitalized with bleeding stomach ulcers than those who don't use these medications.

COMMONLY USED NSAIDS

Generic Name	Brand Name
Ibuprofen	Advil, Motrin
Diclofenac	Voltaren
Naproxen	Anaprox, Naprosyn
Indomethacin	Indocin
Piroxicam	Feldene
Ketoprofen	Orudis

Another commonly prescribed medication is acetaminophen. Tylenol is the most common brand of acetaminophen on the market. The FDA has mandated that all prescription medications, such as Vicodin and Norco, decrease the amount of acetaminophen in their formulations due to studies that show the potential kidney damage acetaminophen can cause. The risk is dose-dependent, beginning at around one hundred pills per year.

Due to the side effects of medications, more people than ever are looking at alternative options. There are excellent alternatives to prescription and over-the-counter medications commonly prescribed post-trauma or surgery. In fact, several supplements on the market today can help decrease the CRP (C-reactive) marker, which can

TESTING FOR CRP

Today there is a simple test to identify whether or not someone is suffering from low-grade chronic inflammation. A CRP (C-reactive protein) test is a blood test performed by physicians and some dentists. Most integrative and functional doctors and nutritionists test for CRP automatically because it is such an important marker today. High levels of CRP are associated with a higher risk of diabetes, periodontal disease, arthritis, hypertension, and obesity, and can indicate an increased risk of heart attack and stroke by as much as 400-800 percent.

I believe everyone should be screened for CRP levels in order to avoid disease by taking a proactive approach to health. CRP levels can be surprisingly high, even in those patients who think they are healthy and exercise regularly. For instance, one of my patients, India, had been a triathlete for many years. Outwardly, she appeared to be in great shape, but she didn't heal well after oral surgery and the area was inflamed for a long time. I checked her CRP and found it to be above 7—levels should register as close to 0 as possible, but normal is around 5.0 mg/L (milligrams per liter). High levels of CRP are not surprising among athletes, especially those that eat a lot of sugar for energy. I recommended a program of anti-inflammatory supplements to her, along with a change in diet to decrease high-glycemic foods when not in competition.

indicate chronic inflammation. These supplements can help decrease chronic inflammation, allowing for faster healing.

CHOOSING THE RIGHT SUPPLEMENTS

In today's market, there is information on nutritional supplementation everywhere. Overwhelming numbers of nutritional supplements line the aisles of any pharmacy or natural food store, the latter of which seem to be popping up on every corner.

"Which one should I take, doctor?" That's a question I often hear from my patients.

Unfortunately, the strict regulation that applies to prescription drugs does not apply to nutritional supplements. The FDA regulates dietary supplements, but there is still a significant amount of adulteration going on, whether intentional by the supplier or unintentional due to the environment the ingredients are grown in.

Oftentimes, suppliers add fillers to certain supplements to enable them to be sold at a lower cost. Supplements such as ginseng root, ginkgo, saw palmetto, CoQ10, black cohosh, and fish oil, are particularly susceptible to fillers. Contamination of these supplements can be biological or chemical, and can range from impurities to lack of absorption ability, so it's important for every batch to be tested. Unfortunately, testing is done mostly by the companies selling the products, so not all the ingredients on the label are accurate.

In 2012, the FDA inspected 361 dietary supplement facilities and found that about 70 percent were not following proper manufacturing practices. Most of the tainted products were in the category of weight loss, sex enhancement, and bodybuilding. For example, many weight loss supplements actually contained diuretics and stimulants. In 2015, thousands of supplements were taken off the shelf at major pharmacies—Walgreens, Target, and GNC—in New York City, because the capsules did not contain the ingredients listed on the label.

Let's talk about probiotics. Approximately four million Americans take supplements of probiotics, which continues to grow exponentially. Most probiotics sitting on supermarket shelves are likely already dead and will have no effect. That's why it is best to go with a reputable company when buying these supplements.

The question then is: How do you know the company has good reputation? Most health care professionals use companies with high-quality products, and it is advisable to follow their recommendations. Here are some of the questions to ask before you start using certain products; these questions can also help if you are researching on your own:

- Does the company carry the Current Good Manufacturing Practices (cGMP) seal?

- Has the company received any warning letters from the FDA?

- Has the company recalled a product in the last five years?

- Does the company regularly test the potency of its products?

Even when you do take reputable dietary supplements, your body may not be absorbing them properly, and a detoxification process may be necessary to clean out the intestinal tract.

When healing, the body needs an optimal level of vitamins, minerals, antioxidants, and other micronutrients. However, when a person is in a diseased state, a lack of nutrients is usually present.

Personalized medicine allows vitamins and minerals to be best customized to each individual's needs. A simple blood or urine test can help determine what supplementation is necessary, and can be provided by nutritionists and integrative doctors.

VITAMINS TO SUPPLEMENT GOOD EATING

I am a true believer in getting most of our vitamins from the food we eat. Unfortunately, it is nearly impossible to do that today. Since farming soils have been nearly depleted of nutrients, the amount of vitamins in fresh food is not what it used to be fifty years ago.

Many patients ask me, "Isn't it enough to take a regular multivitamin?"

Well, the answer is, "no." Most people are actually mineral deficient, not vitamin deficient. Many of the multivitamins out there do not absorb well and they don't contain sufficient minerals, if any at all. If you want to take a multivitamin/mineral supplement, I recommend taking the whole-food-derived formula and make sure it contains minerals.

The reviews about whether or not people should take a daily multivitamin supplement are mixed. In 2002, the *Journal of the American Medical Association* (*JAMA*) published an article by Harvard researchers recommending, "All adults take one multivitamin daily." That recommendation remains standard more than a decade later.

However, taking a multivitamin daily is by no means a replacement of a healthy, whole-food diet. Multivitamins should only supplement the diet. And unfortunately, most multivitamins available to consumers are synthetic, manufactured from wood and petroleum. I prefer vitamins from whole food sources, which means they are more bioavailable.

We have come a long way since the first vitamin was discovered in the early 1900s. The research on the viability of different vitamins is abundant and ongoing. The problem with research in the field is that it is hard to isolate one single nutrient and see what effect it has on the human body. All the nutrients and vitamins must be in balance with enzymes to achieve optimum health and healing. I'll discuss enzymes in-depth later in the chapter.

Research looking at the effect of specific vitamin deficiencies on wound healing has been studied mostly in animals. For instance, research has found that vitamin B5, or pantothenic acid supplementation, can increase the tensile strength of skin scars. Thiamin and vitamin C are essential to normal collagen formation, and are necessary in all healing, whether that is bone, connective tissue, or skin. Vitamin C supplementation of 500 mg per day has been shown to accelerate healing of surgical wounds and pressure sores. Vitamin A and E levels are also important in healing, and deficiency has been shown to slow down recovery.

Vitamin D—Other Issues with Deficiencies

In chapter 2, I talked about sunlight as a natural source of vitamin D. Vitamin D has gotten a lot of attention in the last few years. Every month, it seems, I read about a new study on vitamin D in a nutritional magazine. It turns out that the majority of people, even people living in Southern California where there is lots of sunshine, are deficient in this very important nutrient. Prior to oral surgery, I ask many of my patients if they know their vitamin D level. Since we are in Southern California, a common response is: "I'm sure my vitamin D is fine." But just living in a place with plenty of sunshine is no guarantee—I spend a lot of time outdoors on weekends, and even I have been deficient.

Studies in recent years show the role of vitamin D in systemic health and oral health. Systemically, vitamin D deficiency increases the risk for osteoporosis, high blood pressure, heart problems, allergies, colds and flu, and poor mental health. Studies have also shown that deficiencies of vitamin D contribute to an increased rate of osteo-porosis, Alzheimer's disease, and hair loss. In oral health, vitamin D deficiencies increase the risk of infection, periodontitis, cavities, and failed dental implants. In a recent study involving 9,700 patients, it was concluded that deficiencies were associated with increased rates of infection, sepsis, and mortality.

Vitamin D has also been shown to play a vital role in cancer treatment. It modulates cell growth, immune function, and reduces inflammation. It can activate certain genes, which regulate cell proliferation, division, and turnover. Vitamin D likewise plays a key role in bone mineral density by promoting adequate calcium absorption in the intestines, and by maintaining adequate levels of calcium and phosphate in the body for bone mineralization. This is especially important during dental implant osseointegration, which is the attachment of jawbone to the implant. Vitamin D is necessary for bone remodeling and the proper functioning of osteoblasts and osteoclasts, which are the cells that tear down and rebuild bone as part of the natural function of the body.

The recommended daily dose of vitamin D has gone from 600 IU (international units) in 1997 to 4,000 IU today. How can you get more vitamin D without supplementation? In addition to a daily dose of sunshine, nutritional sources of vitamin D include mushrooms, eggs, and fish, such as salmon and sardines.

The best way to check that your vitamin D level is optimum is with a blood test. Several laboratories offer testing via a quick nick of the finger. Patients can also order a kit directly from the lab, and perform the test in the comfort of their home. The test is known as a dry blood spot, which involves placing the drop of blood on a piece of test paper and allowing it to dry before sending in to a lab. See your physician or nutritionist to recommend the right dose to keep your vitamin D at optimum levels.

MINERALS—THE PRIMARY DEFICIENCY

Without minerals, vitamins cannot function properly, yet most people are deficient in minerals. Weston Price, DDS, who researched the effects of diet in the early 1900s, reported that tribal people living in other areas of the world ate four times more minerals in their diet than the US population did in the 1930s.

Today, that gap is likely even bigger due to rampant soil depletion of minerals through modern farming methods, along with the use of pesticides and chemicals used to increase crop yields. That process started in the early 1900s, and studies have shown that soils have since depleted 30 to 80 percent of essential minerals.

Refinement of foods also depletes minerals. For example, white flour-processing decreases the mineral content in breads and pastas by 80 to 90 percent. Some medications can partially block the absorptions of certain minerals, so patients taking medications can become more deficient. In fact, data from the National Institutes of Health shows that most people do not meet the recommended daily allowance of many minerals. Despite the data, many health care practitioners still overlook the importance of mineral supplementation.

Minerals not only support healthy bones and teeth, but also play a key role in proper blood formation, cellular energy, nerve function, detoxification, and a healthy immune system. During healing, if minerals are deficient, cell regeneration does not occur and chronic disease sets in. For instance, a deficiency in zinc can leave the body more prone to infections.

When it comes to oral surgery and bone healing of the jaw, patients often ask me if more calcium will help their healing. Calcium on its own, if not taken in conjunction with vitamin D, magnesium, and boron, will not be absorbed properly—most of it will end up going down the drain. Due to the interconnection of minerals in their function, I recommend taking a multi-mineral supplement, not just one individual supplement.

My favorite form of mineral supplementation is in liquid form or clay-based tablet. Supplementation should be taken every day to promote health, and it is especially important during healing. The absorption of minerals also depends on their constitution. For example, calcium carbonate is not as readily absorbed as calcium citrate. A formulation of plant-based calcium is ideal, as it is more bioavailable for absorption via the intestinal tract.[4]

In humans and animals, minerals are primarily concentrated in the bones and account for about 4 to 5 percent of total body weight. Minerals are classified as macrominerals and trace elements, depending on the quantity present in our body. Calcium, magnesium, phosphorus, potassium, chloride, sodium, and sulphur are the primary macrominerals. Trace elements are boron, cobalt, chromium, copper, iodine, iron, manganese, molybdenum, nickel, silicon, selenium, silicon, tin, zinc, and vanadium, which are essential

---

4   More information about the benefits of minerals can be found in the book, *Mineral Miracle*, by Shari Lieberman, Ph.D. and Alan Xenakis, M.D.

to health. However, the trace mineral list doesn't stop there; more are being discovered even today. Let me share a bit more about some of the macrominerals and trace minerals.

Macrominerals

Calcium is the most abundant mineral in the body. Although 99 percent of calcium is in the bones, some of it is used for blood clotting and proper cell division during healing. During times of growth and healing, the need for calcium increases. Common signs of calcium deficiency are: anxiety, insomnia, muscle cramping, twitching, and brittle, white-spotted nails. Long-term calcium deficiency results in osteopenia (low bone density) and eventually osteoporosis, which is when the bones weaken and can break easier.

Magnesium, abundant in bones and muscles, is needed for energy production in repair of cells during healing. More than 70 percent of the population in the United States is magnesium deficient. Signs of magnesium deficiency are high blood pressure, irregular heartbeat, memory problems, muscle spasms, and cramping in the hands. Good sources of magnesium are green vegetables, beans, and seafood.

Phosphorus is the second most abundant mineral in the body. It is primarily found in the hydroxyapatite structure of bones and teeth. Phosphorus deficiency is rare, however, it can happen in someone who is vegetarian. Overuse of antacid can also block mineral absorption, and may cause a deficiency. A simple switch from antacids to digestive enzymes with a meal can restore mineral absorption. Foods rich in protein are typically rich in phosphorus.

Potassium and **chloride**, along with **sodium**, are essential electrolytes, which allow the conduction of the electrical stimuli from cell to cell. Deficiency in potassium is common, particularly among the elderly and those suffering from chronic diseases that take medication. Symptoms of potassium deficiency include fatigue, high blood pressure, irregular heartbeat, slow wound healing, and nervous problems.

Sulfur is necessary for the formation and repair of collagen. It is an essential component in cellular and brain function, as well as oxygen utilization. It is also an important component in healthy joints, and aids in ridding waste products from cells. Sulfur deficiencies manifest results of eczema, other skin problems, along with brittle hair and nails. It is found in eggs, onions, and cruciferous vegetables, like broccoli.

Trace Elements

Boron is important in bone mineralization and facilitates calcium absorption. It may also play a role in cellular membrane formation. Boron is found in beans, nuts, and vegetables.

Chromium aids in glucose metabolism. Deficiency is associated with neuropathy and insulin resistance. It is a recommended supplement for diabetic patients. Dietary sources are grains, nuts, potatoes, and seafood.

Cobalt is a trace mineral that assists in the proper function of vitamin B12. It aids in nerve conduction and the proper functioning of red blood cells. A cobalt deficiency is similar to a B12 deficiency, manifesting in anemia, loss of appetite, fatigue, and nerve problems.

Copper is an important mineral in healing and recovery. It helps produce collagen and maintain healthy red blood cells. In recent years, copper deficiency has been shown to play a role in many chronic illnesses, including cancer. Taking too much zinc will inhibit copper absorption. In healing, it activates many enzymatic reactions and is a potent antioxidant. Copper deficiency is fairly common and symptoms manifest as fatigue, swelling, anemia, and damaged blood vessels. Copper is found in shellfish, nuts, and seeds.

Iodine is an essential food for the thyroid gland. Thyroid hormones are essential in energy production, circulation, and metabolism. Iodine supplementation is vital to good health. In the United States, iodine deficiency is rampant and millions of people are affected. Swelling of the thyroid at the base of the neck can be a sign of iodine deficiency. Common symptoms are fatigue, depression, and weight gain. If you don't eat fish and iodized salt, most likely you are deficient in iodine. Most people today are switching to sea salt, because it is a healthier salt, which I highly recommend. However, that means adding iodine back into the diet. Certain vegetables eaten raw, such as cabbage, kale, spinach, and cauliflower can block the uptake of iodine. Iodine drops can be purchased at the health food store, and can be taken on a daily basis. Fish, shellfish, and algae are good sources of iodine.

Iron is an important mineral in healing, because of its role in the immune system function and energy production. Its primary role is to transport oxygen to the tissues and keep the red blood cells healthy. Women and the elderly are prone to iron deficiency, which compromises their immune system to fight against infection. Common iron deficiency symptoms are dizziness, headaches, sleep problems, and fatigue.

Manganese is required for the production of collagen, fatty-acid synthesis, and many other cellular functions. It is also found in the pituitary gland. During healing of bone fractures and connective tissue, the requirement for manganese increases. Symptoms of deficiency are memory loss, poor muscle coordination and weakness, and dizziness. Dietary sources are nuts, grains, and tea.

Molybdenum participates in several enzymatic functions, and it pairs up with iron, copper, and sulfur metabolism. A deficiency in molybdenum manifests as neurocognitive problems, such as irritability. It is found in dairy, grains, and legumes.

Nickel plays a role in the formation of proteins and it is mainly found in RNA, a molecule inside cells. Supplementation is not necessary, as deficiency is relatively rare. Nickel is commonly found in most plant-based foods.

Selenium testing is getting quite a lot of attention in the recent years. Selenium is a key part of the immune system. It acts as an antioxidant and has been shown to have anticancer properties. It aids the body in detoxification from heavy metals and toxins. Many people are selenium deficient, but selenium can be easily replenished by eating whole grains and Brazil nuts.

Silicon aids in detoxification of cells. During healing, silicon helps eliminate toxins that gather at the site, helping to prevent stagnation and swelling. Without sufficient silicon, tissues respond slowly when repairing and healing. Signs of silicon deficiency include brittle nails, tendonitis, and osteoporosis.

Strontium is important in the structural part of the cell. It is a key component of healthy bones and teeth.

Tin is found in almost all tissues, and it is thought to be useful in intracellular activity, but the exact mechanism is unknown.

Vanadium is widely found in the human body, especially in teeth bones and fatty tissues. It aids in enzymatic reactions. Dietary sources are shellfish, mushrooms, and spices, such as black pepper.

Zinc plays a major role in healing. It is the catalyst for hundreds of enzymatic reactions and a powerful antioxidant that aids in detoxification. It is also a key component of the immune system. Zinc is found in the membrane and inside every cell. It helps maintain a balanced level of vitamin A. Zinc deficiency symptoms include susceptibility to infections, fatigue, loss of appetite, prostate problems, and hair loss.

OMEGA-3 FATTY ACIDS

Fish oil has invaded the market. Due to the enormous amount to research, almost everyone is taking this supplement. Omega-3 oils play a major role in the membrane fluidity of cells. These oils have been shown to have an anti-inflammatory effect, decrease blood pressure and depression, joint pain, and improve cardiovascular health, reducing the risk of stroke and heart attack. When it comes to recovery from brain injuries, Omega-3 has shown amazing results.

Not all Omega-3 supplements on the market are created equal. Some of the fish oil supplements may have a higher level of mercury and other toxins. It is good to know the manufacturer you choose. When in doubt, ask your doctor for a recommendation on which is best.

If you're planning on having surgery, make sure to discontinue any fish oil or Omega-3 formulations two weeks prior to your procedure, as they can cause increased bleeding postoperatively.

ENZYMES AND HEALING

Most people are aware that adequate amounts of vitamins and minerals are needed to survive, and that proteins, carbohydrates, and fats are necessary in the everyday diet.

But most people are unaware how essential enzyme supplementation is to health. When I mention the word enzymes, most people think about digestion. Yes, enzymes help digest foods. Fresh vegetables and fruits, as well as unpasteurized dairy products, contain natural enzymes. However, through the cooking process, all enzymes are destroyed above a temperature of 118 degrees Fahrenheit.

Enzymes are also involved in nearly all processes in the body, including healing. Edward Howell, MD, extensively studied enzyme nutrition in the early to mid-1900s. In his book, *Enzymes for Health and Longevity*, he was the first to acknowledge and present evidence of the role of enzymes in healing from chronic diseases. In recent years, research on enzymes has proven their importance in decreasing inflammation. Enzyme research in the field of cancer is also ongoing and is showing promising results as an adjunct to conventional treatment. Studies have also confirmed the use of enzymes in treating rheumatoid arthritis, osteoarthritis, and sports injuries.

Enzymes are proteins that induce chemical changes in the body without undergoing changes themselves. Enzymes cannot function without vitamins and minerals, which are actually called co-enzymes.

Enzymes are classified into six groups, based on their function: hydrolases, lysases, oxidoreductases, transferases, isomerases, and ligases. Of these, proteases, amylases, and lipases play an important role in post-surgical repair.

Following a surgical procedure or an accident, the tissues that were damaged or injured must be replaced. That happens when an inflammatory reaction sets in and the synthesis for all kinds of proteins increases. Enzymes are necessary for that synthesis. Think of enzymes as the workers who assemble the tissue; and proteins, carbohydrates, and fats as the building blocks. Besides the synthesis of new proteins and activating the immune system, enzymes also break down fiber and clots in the surgical site.

Enzymes are classified into six groups, based on their function: hydrolases, lysases, oxidoreductases, transferases, isomerases, and ligases.

Deficiencies in enzymes can result in a longer period of inflammation and pain. Supplementation with proteolytic enzymes can accelerate healing by up to 50 percent. In fact, several studies have shown that enzymes can have similar effects to nonsteroidal anti-inflammatory drugs, such as ibuprofen. Although nonsteroidal anti-inflammatory drugs relieve pain, they also slow down the tissue repair by suppressing the natural healing response. That's why, if possible, it is best to avoid these pain medications during healing.

Bromelain is a protease enzyme derived from the pineapple stem, which has been getting a lot of attention due to its anti-inflammatory properties. Protease refers to the enzyme's ability to break down proteins and peptides, which are made up amino acids. Several studies looked at bromelain's effectiveness after a wisdom tooth extraction and it was determined to have similar results in decreasing pain and inflammation as NSAIDs, but without the gastrointestinal side effects. The recommended dose is 500 mg three times a day, taken on an empty stomach. People allergic to pineapple should avoid taking bromelain.

Quercetin is an enzyme with anti-inflammatory properties that is extracted from onion. It is found on the market in a supplement form by itself, or in conjunction with bromelain. Studies indicate that oral quercetin is readily absorbed in the bloodstream. Aside from its use as the postsurgical recovery supplement, quercetin is also studied in relation to systemic diseases. The association between dietary quercetin intake and risk of several chronic diseases was studied in 10,054 Finnish men and women. Based on dietary history from the previous year, people with higher quercetin intakes had lower mortality from ischemic heart disease, lower incidence of asthma, and lower risk of developing type 2 diabetes. Men with higher quercetin intakes had a lower prostate cancer risk and lower lung cancer incidence. Several studies also report benefits of quercetin for management of various chronic inflammatory conditions.

One of my patients, Kate, had such severe gum disease that all of her teeth had to be replaced with implants. Since she could not take ibuprofen, I recommended bromelain enzymes postsurgically. A week later, she reported that the enzymes not only helped her mouth, but also decreased the long-time pain she had endured in her hip. This is quite a common experience I hear from patients. Enzymes are an ideal solution to joint pain, but consult a health care practitioner prior to deciding which enzyme formulation is right for you.

Most enzymes today are used for digestive purposes. These can come in the form of plant-based enzymes as well as animal-derived enzymes, such as pancreatin. Proteolytic (protease) enzymes combat bacteria, fungi, and viruses, and also break down fibrin (protein strands) stuck inside arteries, which can lead to vascular disease. Other formulations of enzymes on the market are specifically designed for inflammation reduction and healing. Most anti-inflammatory formulations are plant-based. To be sure, you must check with the manufacturer. If you're taking enzymes for anti-inflammatory purposes, they must be taken on an empty stomach. That way they can be absorbed into the blood, where they can start cleaning up foreign pathogens.

Right now, studies show that, as people age, their enzymes decrease in number and functional ability; the body's enzyme production decreases every year. Symptoms of enzyme deficiency include:

- Heartburn

- Constipation

- Bloating

- Cramping after eating

- Flatulence

Fresh, uncooked, unpasteurized foods (fruits, vegetables, cheese) are full of enzymes, which are released when the food is chewed thoroughly. Unfortunately, the standard American diet consists mostly of cooked, processed foods, devoid of any enzymes. Many people suffer from digestive issues, such as heartburn, and are prescribed antacids. Enzymes work just as well, but with far fewer side effects. Antacids block the absorption of calcium and other minerals and should not be taken on a regular basis.

PROBIOTICS FOR HEALTH

Digestive problems have increased in recent years, not only due to increase in sugary and processed foods, but also due to increase in stressors and the number of prescription medications.

Since the discovery of antibiotics, the medical community has focused on treating infections by wiping out bacteria. This has resulted in a landscape where infections have become resistant to drugs, even in the presence of the strongest antibiotics. According to the Centers for Disease Control and Prevention, twenty-three thousand people die every year from infections that are untouched by antibiotics.

Antibiotics work great when they are not abused. Unfortunately, they are overused and overprescribed. In most parts of the world, such as Europe and Asia, antibiotics are sold over-the-counter. In the United States, they are commonly prescribed for colds, which are viral infections that won't respond to them.

In recent years, research has found that friendly bacteria can actually protect against infections. That has led to exponential growth in the field of probiotics ("pro" meaning "for" and "biotics" meaning "life").

Probiotic supplementation has been shown to be beneficial in battling digestive issues, cold and flu, sinusitis, eczema, yeast infections, chronic fatigue, depression, obesity, and diabetes.

Probiotics are dietary supplements that replenish the beneficial bacteria and produce beneficial substances, such as B12, amino acids, and antimicrobials. Friendly bacteria are necessary for the absorption and breakdown of nutrients in the digestive tract. If the digestive tract is not healthy, either due to constipation or yeast overgrowth, then absorption of the necessary nutrients for healing is stagnated. The digestive tract starts with the mouth, because that is where digestion begins. The mouth, stomach, and intestinal passage hold about two to three pounds of bacteria. People cannot live without these bacteria, and yet many things can affect their well-being including antibiotics, prescription drugs, over-the-counter pain medications (such as NSAIDs), stress, and processed foods.

Here are some ways that we know these little bacteria benefit our bodies:

- Enhance immune function
- Decrease inflammation
- Prevent allergies
- Provide energy by producing B12
- Decrease bloating and constipation
- Help with depression and weight loss

To maintain a healthy digestive tract full of friendly bacteria, I recommend a serving of fermented foods daily: kefir, yogurt, sauerkraut (fermented, not pickled), kimchi, kombucha, miso, or natto. If these don't sound appetizing, not to worry! A daily probiotic capsule will do.

Most people are familiar with the bacteria known as acidophilus, but there are literally hundreds of different species of bacteria lining the digestive system. With the Lactobacillus acidophilus bacteria alone, there are approximately two hundred different strains with different potencies. Of these, less than twenty are the most potent.

When taking a probiotic, look for one with at least ten different kinds of beneficial bacteria. Very few probiotics made by reputable companies can be stored at room temperature, most should be kept refrigerated. A great new drinkable probiotic is Bio-K, with fifty billion probiotics in each dose. Also look for a product that contains at least 2 billion bifidobacterium, which are the major inhabitants and protectors of the large intestine. When they are present in the right amount, disease causing bacteria cannot survive. Bifidobacteria also contribute to the production of B-complex vitamins and assist in liver detoxification.

No single probiotic formula works well for everyone. It is best to start with a lower dosage and increase it, if needed. Side effects are rare, and if they do occur, they tend to be mild gas and loose stool, which are easily reversed by stopping the probiotics.

When taking antibiotics, I recommend a probiotic to be taken in conjunction with your prescription. A probiotic will minimize any unwanted side effects, such as diarrhea and fatigue. Take at least fifty billion cfu two to four hours following the antibiotic, and continue with the probiotic for at least one month.

Chewable probiotics for oral health issues have shown promising results. People who develop ulcers in the mouth, such as canker sores, may lack beneficial bacteria. D.J. Weekes, MD, in the 1980s, reported successful use of chewable tablets of Lactobacillus acidophilus and bulgaricus with several patients who suffered from mouth ulcers. Patients suffering from thrush also found oral probiotics alleviated their symptoms. Thrush, a common ailment of people who wear dentures, appears as a patchy tongue, fiery red roof of the mouth, or soreness at the corners of the mouth. It stems from yeast overgrowth (candida), which can occur in various areas of the body including all the way into the intestinal tract. Candida albicans, a fungus, is typically present in small numbers in healthy individuals. In a moist environment, coupled with a high-sugar diet, there can be an overgrowth of it. The common treatment for candida albican is nystatin. Unfortunately, once the medication ends, the condition sometimes returns. That is why I often recommend chewable probiotics and a low-sugar diet to prevent yeast overgrowth.

Oral probiotic studies have shown it can reduce cavities significantly, by reducing the level of the cavity-causing bacteria, Streptococcus mutans. Lactobacillus species are also beneficial for gingivitis and inflammation. In my practice, chewable probiotics are an essential part of getting the mouth back to health. More than 70 percent of people walking through our doors have oral diseases including periodontal disease, cavities, oral sores/ulcers. They all have one thing in common: a disruption in the biofilm. This can be combatted with chewable probiotics. Oral probiotics can come in the form of lozenges, chewing gum, chewable tablets, powders, liquids, or food, and they taste good. Optimum dosage of oral probiotics is still being researched, but to date the recommendation is one hundred million to one billion per day. The best time to take oral probiotics is after a meal, or at bedtime.

One interesting bacteria to mention is S. salivarius, which has been shown to combat bad breath and to prevent plaque from sticking to the tooth surface. It is currently available in Canada and the United States over-the-counter. No side effects have been seen so far.

MEDICINAL MUSHROOMS

Mushrooms have been used for thousands of years to treat different disease conditions, including cancer. Shamans used the mushrooms attached to trees as powerful medicines. Otzi, the 5,300-year-old ice-age man who was discovered in 1991, amongst the mountains between Austria and Italy, carried with him birch polypore mushrooms, which are known to have antibacterial and anti-parasitic properties.

Mushrooms are high in antioxidants, B vitamins, vitamin D, and minerals, such as selenium, copper, and potassium. All these elements are important for a healthy immune function. Andrew Weil, MD, a leader in integrative medicine, recommends a regular consumption of medicinal mushrooms such as shiitake, to help prevent diseases. Many mushrooms also have the capacity to strengthen the immune system, but some stand out more than others: reishi, chaga, turkey tail, shiitake, to name a few.

There is still much to be learned about the health benefits of mushrooms. The medicinal active compounds in mushrooms are polysaccharides, triterpenes, glycoproteins, and antibiotics.

Polysaccharides have the capacity to activate the immune system and also slow down or stop the growth of tumors.

Ergosterol is a compound present in mushrooms that inhibits proliferation of blood vessels that support tumors. One particular mushroom, Cordyceps sinensis, which grows in the Himalayas as a parasite on caterpillar larvae, is often used for medicinal properties in the Western world. It is a revitalizing supplement that increases the power of the immune system, liver, and kidneys.

Certain mushrooms also produce natural **antibiotics**, which are effective against bacteria, viruses, and parasites. Reishi is Japanese for "divine." In Chinese, the reishi mushroom is called "the tree of life." These mushrooms have a direct antimicrobial effect, and also stimulate the production of immune cells called macrophages. They decrease allergies and histamine release due to their **triterpene** content. Research has also shown that combining different species of mushroom has a greater impact on the immune system.

I have used mushroom supplements to help the immune system fight against tumors. A patient of mine came in with a tumor inside the mouth, which had been removed twice before via conventional surgery. Instead of removing it, we activated the immune system via supplementation with medicinal mushrooms, vitamins, minerals, and local homeopathic injections. After six weeks of treatment, the tumor not only stopped growing in size, but it started to shrink. Six months later, the tumor completely disappeared.

The National Institutes of Health (NIH) is currently conducting research on different medicinal properties of mushrooms. Turkey tail mushrooms are being studied in relation to breast cancer, as an adjunct to a chemotherapy treatment. Results are promising, and show that a combination is more effective in eradicating cancer.

HOMEOPATHIC REMEDIES

Homeopathy can be extremely helpful in alleviating the discomfort associated with healing. It can also aid in treating several acute, as well as chronic conditions.

Homeopathy dates back to the 19th century. The founder of homeopathy is Samuel Hahnemann, a German physician. Hahnemann and his associates tested one hundred different compounds. One of his students, Constantin Hering, who introduced homeopathy in the United States, studied an additional six hundred friend compounds. Today, there are over 1,400 different homeopathic compounds.

Contrary to popular belief, homeopathy is not herbal medicine. Homeopathic remedies are infinitesimal diluted extracts from plants, living organisms, and inorganic compounds, such as minerals. Dating back to the 5th century BC, Hippocrates noted that a toxic condition caused by a certain plant can be reversed by using the same plant in extremely diluted quantities. Hippocrates said: "The same things which caused a disease cure it." For example, Arnica Montana, a plant growing in the mountains, can cause swelling and bruising when ingested. The same plant, if taken in very small dilutions, can reverse bruising and swelling associated with surgical procedures and injuries. Hahnemann also noted that if he gave ipecac to healthy people, it induced nausea and vomiting. However, when patients were suffering from nausea and vomiting, the administration of small therapeutic doses of ipecac caused the symptoms to disappear.

Unlike prescription drugs and medications, homeopathic remedies work with the body, rather than suppressing the symptoms. Conventional medicine works to inhibit and destroy, while homeopathy cooperates with the immune system to eliminate the problem.

There has been extensive research in the field of homeopathy since the 19th century. In Europe, homeopathy is taught in medical schools, and is widely practiced by physicians. In France, about one third of all physicians use homeopathy as part of their regular practice. Because of its safe history, homeopathic remedies are found over-the-counter. However, it is best to consult a homeopath for maximum effectiveness of these remedies.

Homeopathic formulations can come in the form of tinctures dissolved in alcohol, or in the form of pellets, which are sugar-based. I do not use the tinctures for patients with alcohol addiction, because they contain up to 60 percent alcohol. The pellets are intended to be placed under the tongue and dissolved in the saliva. Unfortunately, sugar-based pellets may cause cavities if used several times a day, and especially at night, when the mouth is driest and more prone to cavities.

Alan, one of my patients, was using Gelsemium in the evening to help him fall asleep. He left the sugary pellets underneath his tongue as he fell asleep. After six months of taking the pellets, he came in for his dental exam, only to find that all his lower front teeth were decayed—one even needed to be replaced with an implant.

There are no known interactions between homeopathic remedies and any prescription drugs. Here are some of the remedies I commonly use to treat people who have small trauma, bruises and wounds, which are common in my clinical practice. These homeopathic remedies can be used alone or combined with analgesics:

Symptom	Homeopathic Remedy
Edema from acute trauma	Apis mellifica 15c
Pain	Arnica montana 9c
Hematoma, bruising	Arnica montana 9c
Inflammation	Bryonia alba 9c
Nerve trauma	Hypericum perforatum 15c
Post-concussion headache and dizziness	Natrum sulphuricum 15c
Slow healing bone fracture, dental implants	Calcarea phosphorica 6c
Mouth ulcers, burning	Borax 9c
Generalized gingival ulcers	Mercurius corrosivus 15c
Bleeding ulcer (at corners of the mouth)	Nitricum acidum 9c
Nausea	Nux vomica 6c
Anxiety	Gelsemium sempervirens 15c
Fever, facial redness and swelling	Belladonna 9c

Ulcers or canker sores in the mouth, are common following dental treatment. They can be very painful and conventional remedies do not exist to treat the problems. Homeopathy offers pain relief and can help stop the progression of sores. With canker sores, treatment should be started as soon as the symptoms appear in order to be most effective.

Pre and Post-Operative Homeopathy

Many patients suffer from anxiety prior to dental or medical procedures. Anxiety can cause stress, which slows healing postsurgically. Gelsemium 15c or 30c taken the day before a procedure is recommended to decrease anxiety and to help with falling asleep.

Arnica montana is widely used by many plastic surgeons to minimize bleeding, swelling, and pain following a surgical procedure. I recommend patients start taking arnica montana the morning of any surgical procedure, and continue for one week after. Arnica montana limits hemorrhaging, and speeds absorption of the bruises and edema caused by surgical procedures. Many of my patients choose to take Arnica montana instead of NSAIDs.

Another homeopathic remedy is Staphysagria 5c, which accelerates the closing of wounds caused during surgery. It can be taken for two weeks following surgery.

Because no one has been able to prove scientifically how homeopathy works in the body, Western medicine has not fully embraced homeopathy. Since it is safe and relatively inexpensive, the only risk is that the treatment may not work. Sometimes, however, symptoms get worse before they get better, which is a part of treatment.

SIDE EFFECTS AND INTERACTIONS
OF SUPPLEMENTS

As with other medications, natural supplements can have side effects. These are important to know, especially if scheduled for surgery. Mixing prescription and over-the-counter medications with dietary supplements can also endanger your health.

As a health practitioner, I find that most patients do not list their supplements on their medical history form. An even bigger problem is that most medical and dental forms do not specifically ask to list the supplements that are being taken on a daily basis. One study conducted at Veterans Administration hospitals shows that only 28 percent of patients taking nutritional supplements tell their doctors about what they are taking. Even if you are not asked, tell your doctor what dietary supplements you are taking. There are certain supplements that can increase the power of certain medications and raise their toxicity in the body.

The five most common natural supplements that can potentially interact with medications are: garlic, valerian, kava, gingko, and St. John's wort, according to a large study done at the Mayo Clinic. If you are taking any of these supplements and also taking medications, make sure you check with your pharmacist for any problems that could arise.

SUPPLEMENTS THAT CAUSE BLOOD THINNING INCLUDE:

- Omega-3 (fish or flax seed oil)
- Garlic
- Gingko
- Ginseng
- Red yeast rice
- Vitamin E

Discontinue any of these supplements ten to fourteen days prior to any surgical procedure, as they may cause increased bleeding and an inability to stop the bleeding post-surgically.

The four most common prescription medications to interact with nutritional supplements are: blood-thinning medications, sedatives, antidepressants, and antidiabetic agents.

The following table lists some of the medication-supplement interactions that are most common:

Drug	Supplement	Side-effects
Aspirin, Ibuprofen	Gingko biloba, evening primrose, or EPO	Blood thinning, increased bleeding when injured/surgery
Benzodiazepines – (such as Halcion, Ativan, Xanax)	Valerian, kava	Increased drowsiness and sedation
Benzodiazepines – (such as Halcion, Ativan, Xanax)	St. John's wort	Reduced sedation effect
Clarythromycin, Azythromicin, Erythromycin, Clyndamycin	St. John's wort	Reduced effectiveness of antibiotic
Codeine, Vicodin, Percocet, Norco	St. John's wort, valerian	Increased analgesic effect
Diphenhydramine (Benadryl)	Valerian, kava	Increased sedative effect
Doxycycline, tetracycline	Calcium, St. John's wort	Decreased absorption of doxycycline
Prednisone	St. John's wort	Decreased effectiveness
Zolpidem (Ambien), Zaleplon (Sonata)	St. John's wort	Decreased effectiveness
Zolpidem (Ambien), Zaleplon (Sonata)	Valerian, kava	Increased sedative effect

Some supplements get eliminated from your body faster than others, and some—such as St. John's wort and kava—may take up to four days to clear the body. If you are taking an oral sedative prior to a dental or medical visit, discontinue St. John's wort or kava four days prior to your visit. Gingko, evening primrose, and valerian can be discontinued twenty-four hours prior to the appointment, because they can clear the body at a faster rate.

There's an overwhelming amount of research that continues to be done on multiple forms of supplementation. Not just vitamins and minerals, but also medicinal mushrooms, homeopathics, and probiotics. But all the vitamins in the world won't help in the presence of dehydration. Nothing can substitute for water.

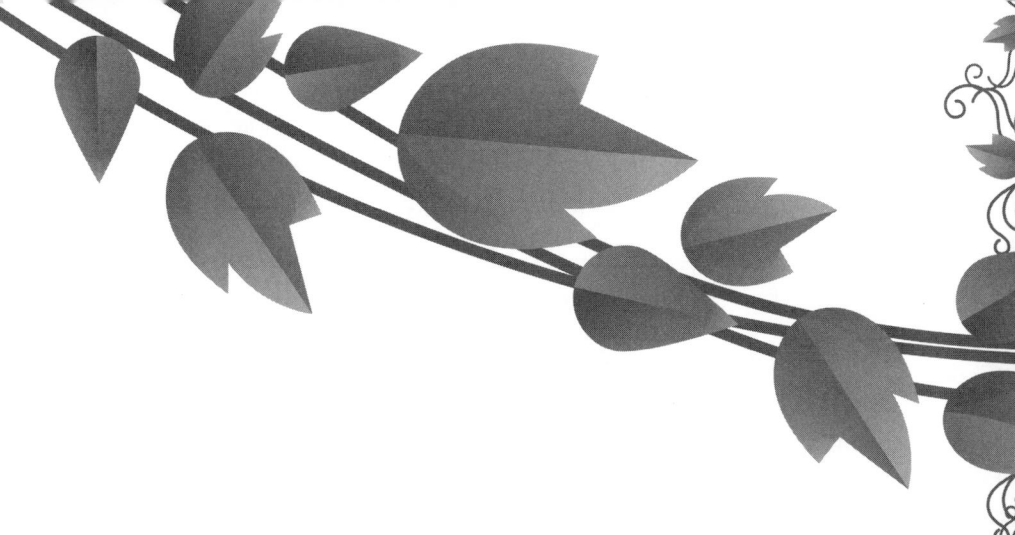

CHAPTER 8

HEALING WITH WATER

My first discovery of the healing power of water was as a young girl, when my mom took me with her on a trip to a balneotherapeutic resort in Romania, Olanesti. The resort ranks first among resorts in Romania in terms of number of mineral springs, their total daily flow, composition, concentration, and variety of minerals in the water. The healing waters are used for drinking as well as bathing, as minerals can be absorbed through the skin. My mom had some digestive issues, which significantly improved after drinking the prescribed water every day. These hot springs are said to increase circulation, which stimulates detoxification and primes the immune system. Stories of these healing hot springs date back to Roman times.

It is estimated that 80 percent of Americans are chronically dehydrated. Dehydration causes the blood cells to become sticky and unable to function properly. When a person is dehydrated, there is an inadequate transfer of oxygen molecules and cellular functions slow down. Scientists have proven that enzymes and proteins within the cells are more efficient when properly hydrated.

There has been extensive research on how better hydration improves the function of the immune system to decrease infection and depression, as well as improve sleep. Water is also necessary for strong bone formation, elevated energy levels, and the prevention of blood clots. Some studies have shown that cognitive functions decrease, even when slightly dehydrated. The human body is made up of mostly water and at 85 to 90 percent, and the brain has the highest water percentage of all the organs.

Water is the key to life; without water humans cannot survive. Every cell in the body has its own ocean within, where all the cellular functions take place. If there is a lack of water, then the water within every cell becomes more viscous, full of toxins, and more difficult to navigate.

TODAY'S WATER CONTROVERSY

So how much water should a person drink? There is still a lot of controversy on the subject. The "eight glasses of water per day" rule never made sense to me, as the theory of unanimity does not apply here. Furthermore, there's no evidence in the research to back a theory that we often read about in health magazines.

How much water a person should drink depends on five things: body weight, activity levels, diet, where you live (hot or cold climate), and how many toxins need to be eliminated. A five-foot-tall, eighty-year-old need not drink the same amount of water as a seven-foot-tall thirty-year-old athlete; their different weights and lifestyles require different levels of water consumption. My eighty-year-old patient may do fine with five to six glasses of water, whereas a professional athlete may need two to three liters of water, depending on how much he or she sweats during physical activity.

A person eating a diet full of vegetables and fruits can get 50 to 70 percent of their daily water from their diet; they won't require as much additional water as someone eating processed, dense foods, such as bread, grains, cookies, and sandwiches. Someone living in a tropical climate by the beach will need more water than someone of the same weight living in a cool climate, because the body uses water to keep its temperature cooler in hotter climates.

Each person should assess how much water they need on an individual basis. Many people drink water only when they are thirsty, but thirst level is not a good measure of determining when to drink. Age, disease, and cold temperature can diminish thirst level, even though dehydration still persists. Furthermore, if someone has been chronically dehydrated for years, they may not have a healthy thirst function anymore.

The best way to assess your level of dehydration is by assessing morning urine color. A dark-colored urine indicates moderate to severe dehydration. If the urine has no color, you may be drinking too much water. Ideally, it should be a pale yellow color. There are other, more complicated ways to assess hydration levels including a 24-hour water input/output, and plasma and urine osmolarity tests.

It is also good to understand how the body expels toxins, even without having a deep knowledge of the physiology of wound healing. During the healing process, many byproducts must be eliminated, and the requirement for water increases. At the site of any injury, an acidic environment surrounds the area, and it is important to keep hydrated in order to speed up recovery and neutralize the acids.

WATER—SO MANY CHOICES

Some patients tell me they only drink water when they are thirsty, yet by that time, their body has already become dehydrated. Instead, it is imperative that water be consumed before the sensation of thirst is felt.

Especially for elderly people, drinking water before thirst sets in is crucial because, as people age, they lose their perception of thirst. A study in the elderly shows that even after a day of water deprivation, patients still experienced no thirst.

The usage of water as a treatment for illnesses has historical context. It was the focus of a doctor, Fereydoon Batmangelidj, MD, who, while working in a prison for a few years treated prisoners' peptic ulcers by having them drink two glasses of water. He was able to successfully treat over three thousand patients using water, a breakthrough that led him to use water to treat several different diseases.

Today, it may become difficult to choose which water is best to drink: super water, antioxidant water, ultra-purified, with added electrolytes—there are a plethora of choices on the market, all bottled and ready to go.

Alkaline Water

Alkaline water has been in circulation for ages. Most spring water at the source is alkaline, and, in my opinion, is the best water for human consumption. As a child in Romania, my family and I used to drive to a local spring to guzzle fresh water from the mountain. At the time, I did not understand why it was so delicious, or why I yearned for it constantly. Now it is clear to me—it was alkaline, but also structured water.

Structured water has more energy, because the water molecules are connected in an organized fashion. Structured water can be found in both rain and spring-water sources. Structured water also has physiological benefits, as human cells more easily absorb it. A fascinating experiment was conducted to prove these benefits. A patient with dehydrated and irregularly shaped blood cells was given two glasses of structured water. Within thirty minutes, the cells became visibly plump and hydrated when observed under a microscope. I thought it would be impossible to find such water in Los Angeles, where I am located. However, the website www.findaspring.com has information about springs all over the world, many of which may contain structured water. Imagine my surprise when I found a spring in the middle of the city, one that has been around since Native Americans populated the area. Big Bear Lake, east of the city, even contains springs that are accessible to the public and are entirely free of cost.

There are several systems on the market that alkalinize water for therapeutic purposes. But, although it is generally better for us, alkaline therapeutic water should not be consumed every day as it could shift your body's physiological balance into an alkaline pH, leading to adverse effects on the cells. The cells require a pH of around 6.8-7.2. I recommend everyone to test their body pH on a regular basis, first thing in the morning through saliva using litmus strips. While many patients may ask if a blood test is more accurate, that is not the case; the body maintains a constant blood pH of 7.4, so blood tests do not give an accurate depiction of the pH level of cells. Those with an acidic salivary pH can benefit from drinking alkaline water, as it can shift after only a few days of consumption.

Filtered Water

Tap water in Los Angeles, like in most urban domains, is processed and treated with chemicals. I recommend obtaining a full analysis of the water coming out of your faucet. There are many companies today that can test your tap water, or you can do it yourself by purchasing a kit and sending it to a lab for results. Some water delivery companies offer the service for free. Color, taste, and smell can give you a superficial assessment of the water quality in your town. However, that will not inform you of all the chemicals that could be present, for example, pesticide runoff from area fields. Cloudy water may indicate bacterial contamination, metallic taste can indicate high levels of iron, and a rotten smell can indicate high levels of sulfur. Some mountain regions have good quality water, but most city water should be filtered.

I believe it is best to filter not only the water that you drink, but the water in which you bathe as well, and a house-water filtration system can take care of both. When you shower or bathe, your skin absorbs water. If a filter is not installed, the human body actually takes its place as a filtration system. Do you want to be a filter for chlorine and other chemicals?

An easy and inexpensive way to filter the water is with an activated charcoal filter, which can filter out pesticides, insecticide, PCBs, heavy metals, asbestos, and volatile organic chemicals (VOC). Oftentimes, activated charcoal systems come with an additional filter for chloride, fluoride, nitrates, and other soluble minerals.

Reverse osmosis water filtering systems are the most effective at removing impurities, including bacteria, parasites, and fungus. However, they also remove all minerals in the water. When that happens, minerals should be reintroduced into the water after the process of reverse osmosis has taken place, or you risk a mineral deficiency. Liquid drops of trace mineral should be added to the water to prevent potential deficiencies.

Bottled water is also a great option for hydration, and is ubiquitous today. While it allows a person to hydrate easily, you should also understand what lies behind the multitude of packaging. The most hydrating, best water to drink, in my opinion, is spring water or artesian water. The less processed, the better it is for the body. It is best to purchase glass bottles instead of plastic to avoid ingesting bisphenol-A (BPA), a carcinogenic chemical that can leach out of plastic bottles, especially when exposed to heat. If you can taste the plastic in the water, do not drink it. It is toxic at that point.

A few years back, when the well-known singer Sheryl Crow contracted breast cancer, it was reported that plastic water bottles may have been the culprit; she used to buy whole cases of water and keep them in her car, even through the hot days of summer. Harmful elements have been shown to leach from plastic bottles into the water as the temperature rises. Doctors discovered plastic residues in her cancerous tumors, which may have come from the heated plastic in the water bottle.

It is also good to know where the bottled water comes from. Some of my favorite locations are Hawaii, Fiji, or Norway. Additionally, try to avoid water that is processed, because it is generally acidic, which can be detrimental during injury or illness. During healing, cells release waste, which tends to be acidic, causing inflammation. Drinking alkaline water can help maintain balance in our bodies. But be careful, some brands of bottled water I've tested on the market can be inconsistent. It is advisable to get a pH meter or pH testing strips and verify the claims on any alkaline water bottle you purchase.

A patient of mine, Patty, is an example of how imperative it is to stay hydrated. She was suffering from generalized periodontal disease, depression, fatigue, diverticulitis (digestive tract inflammation), and neck pain, among other maladies. When I asked Patty about her water consumption, she claimed that she did not drink water, because she did not like the taste. But without it, her body was unable to heal.

To encourage her to drink more, I suggested adding some of her favorite herbs to water at night, which she could then consume the following morning on an empty stomach. After a short time, she began to feel better and experienced elevated levels of energy. Of course, her functional physician and I had more work to complete to help her arrive in a state of optimum healing, but hydrating her body was the key to unlocking her healing potential.

MAKE WATER FUN TO DRINK

If you don't like the taste of plain water, simply add some flavor. At my house, I keep a four-liter jar of water in which I place either herbs, vegetables, fruits, or essential oils: rosemary or mint from my garden, slices of peach, apple, cucumber, or orange essential oil. In a few hours, the flavors are infused into the water, leaving it with a delicious and satisfying taste. Be creative and have fun with it! I also recommend adding a pinch of sea salt or Himalayan salt to give the water minerals that are essential to healing in the human body.

Oxygenated Water

Oxygenated water made its debut several years back, claiming that there's a higher content of oxygen, tested by an independent lab. Although that statement is true, several studies have been conducted to show that, in the short-term, oxygenated water activates the immune system—oxygen radicals can be seen in the blood for sixty minutes after drinking oxygenated water. However, after twenty-one days of drinking oxygenated water, no effect was seen. The problem with the water is that it is difficult to know how stable the extra oxygen in the water actually is. After sitting on the shelf for some time, you might be purchasing just distilled water.

Ozonated Water

Ozone is composed of three molecules of oxygen bound together in comparison to pure oxygen, which is only two molecules bound together. Ozone molecules are not very stable—they only last eighteen to forty hours—so ozonated water cannot be bottled. In chapter 4, I talked about home units for ozonating water. Ozonating your drinking water can remove bacteria, viruses, parasites, or fungi. Ozonated water works well when applied topically to disinfect wounds and burns, and it makes a great, all-natural mouthwash in dentistry. The ozone gas is bubbled into the water for at least ten minutes per half a quart of water, but it has a short half-life and should be consumed shortly after it is made. Within twenty-four hours, the water will lose 50 percent of the ozone injected into it. However, the shelf-life can be prolonged with refrigeration.

There are numerous studies the confirm the benefits of ozonated water. A review article in the *Journal of Contemporary Dental Practice*, stated that: "It can be used for the treatment of alveolitis (jaw infections post extractions) as a replacement for antibiotic therapy, as a mouthwash for reducing the oral microflora, as well as the adherence of microorganisms to tooth surfaces." When compared to a bleach solution, which is toxic to the cells, ozonated water enhanced the cells' function and viability with the same antibacterial effect.

Ionized Water

Water ionization technology comes from Japan. It is an attempt to replicate mountain spring water. Ionization simply means to lose or gain an electron.

Ionized water contains powerful antioxidants, which aid in healing when an excess number of free radicals are being released. Ionized water has been useful for the treatment of diabetes, intestinal problems, liver toxicity, and even cancer. Most chronic diseases are caused by an acidic environment, and drinking ionized water can help reverse the symptoms in most cases. More studies are needed to confirm the benefits of ionized water. What is known is that ionized water does provide the body with extra oxygenation.

When you are starting out drinking alkaline ionized water, begin with only one glass per day, as it can have a detoxifying effect and you may feel like you are coming down with a cold.

Water ionizers separate alkaline from acidic water. While alkaline water is for drinking, acidic water is for detoxifying open wounds. Ionized water lasts approximately eighteen to twenty hours, about the same as ozonated water.

Alkaline ionized water is different than plain alkaline water. Ionization is done by electrolysis, which creates an electromagnetic field to manipulate water molecules. Electrolysis releases negatively charged ions, which can scavenge positively charged bacteria and toxins in your intestinal tract.

Acidic ionized water has been studied in the medical field, as well as the food industry for its ability to inactivate disease-causing bacteria, such as E. coli and Staphylococcus aureus. It is an effective disinfectant, without the side-effects of chemicals.

THE DANGERS OF DRY MOUTH

Dry mouth is another condition I see increasing in frequency in my patients, especially in those patients that have had radiation or chemotherapy, or who have been taking several medications, such as antidepressants and ADHD drugs.

The average American takes three types of medications daily, which are metabolized and removed by the liver and the kidneys. Those organs require a sufficient amount of water to eliminate the toxins left behind from medications. When taking any type of medications, be sure to drink more water than normal to flush out the liver and kidneys.

Dry mouth is not a good indication of dehydration. The human body can be severely dehydrated and not experience dry mouth. When dry mouth occurs, some of the delicate processes of the body have already begun to shut down due to dehydration.

Other signs of dehydration include flaky skin, constipation , dry eyes, fatigue, and stiff muscles and joints. Some even believe that many diseases such as asthma, cancer, and autoimmune diseases are due to long-term and persistent dehydration.

Dry mouth occurs because there is not enough saliva being produced. Serious dental consequences can occur if dry mouth becomes chronic. Recently, I treated a forty-three-year-old patient, Bradley, who suffered from dry mouth from chemotherapy and anti-depressant medications. Over the course of only a couple of years, he lost most of his teeth due to cavities. When there isn't enough saliva to mineralize, the teeth get brittle and cannot withstand normal chewing forces. Rampant decay with soft teeth is seen in patients with a dry mouth, as saliva also has antibacterial properties.

If you suffer from dry mouth, daily trays using a calcium phosphate mineral paste, such as an MI Paste, is recommended to prevent cavities. Unfortunately, Bradley came to us too late, and his teeth were replaced with dental implants because they could not be saved.

HYDRATING ALTERNATIVES
TO DRINKING WATER

Many patients wonder what may be consumed in place of water to achieve ideal hydration. Water is best, of course. However, I also recommend herbal teas, mineral water, coconut water, vegetable broths, and bone and fish broths. Caffeinated beverages such as black tea and coffee can be dehydrating, and should not be the basis of anyone's daily fluid intake. Fruit juices are not a good way to stay hydrated; in fact, they should be avoided because they often contain too much sugar.

Fruits should only be eaten whole and in small amounts. The effect of the fiber in fruit slows down the sugar intake, preventing a sugar spike that is common after drinking juice. In spite of that, juicing places have sprouted up all over the United States, especially in Los Angeles. During healing, certain juices can provide much-needed vitamins and minerals. Vegetables and fruits contain structured water, which makes them more absorbable in the intestinal tract. Healing juices are composed of 80-90 percent vegetables, with the remaining percentage composed of fruit for a little bit of sweetness. Vegetable juice on its own, without fruit, is far healthier, as it contains less sugar—although for most people, it is less tolerable. The bulk of any juice should consist of cucumber or celery, which have great electrolytes to replenish the loss of blood from an injury.

Any vegetable can be juiced. I especially recommend the green ones, such as kale, parsley, and wheatgrass, which contain a lot of minerals. Caution should be taken with vegetables such as carrots and beets, which have high levels of sugar. Limit any juices to no more than one beet or one carrot per day. I've included some of my favorite juicing recipes for healing at the back of the book.

Sodas, even the diet variety, are one of the worst options for hydration. The acidity alone is toxic to the body's cells, and most sodas contain chemicals and corn syrups that can erode tooth enamel and cause internal harm to the body. Instead, substituting water for soda can help prevent irreparable damage. One option is to replace soda with mineral water combined with an ounce of fresh orange juice and some stevia or monkfruit drops. Be aware that soda water and mineral water are not the same things; soda water is still acidic compared to mineral water. Many companies post the acidity levels on the label of a bottle of soda so you don't have to measure it at home.

As I mentioned earlier, water is absorbed through the skin, so another way to achieve hydration is through bathing. The skin is the body's largest organ and its powerful role in maintaining internal balance is often underestimated. Baths can add about 20 percent hydration through the skin. But in today's busy world, most people take a quick shower, which doesn't give the skin enough time to absorb water. I encourage you to incorporate twenty-minute baths in your weekly ritual. One therapeutic bath a week can release toxins, mineralize the body, and hydrate the cells. This can be especially useful when preparing for surgery. To make the bath water therapeutic, I recommend adding sea salts, Epsom salts, essential oils, seaweed, or even clay.

Hydration is a key factor in disease prevention and wellness and should be maintained consistently throughout your entire life. Water is essential and is one of the most important nutrients in the human body.

CONCLUSION

●●

C ongratulations! You have completed your journey of learning ways to repair, rebuild, and renew naturally! Now you are on the path to better health and healing.

Here's a summary list for you to heal up. Consider it like a *daily* checklist to start at least two weeks before any planned surgical procedure.

1. **EAT YOUR VEGGIES.** Eat a rainbow of colors on your plate as often as possible. This will help you get those phytonutrients and antioxidants essential for healing and recovery.

2. **PICK GOOD FATS.** Such as avocadoes, coconut, and olive oils. These are essential for your cells, nerves, and hormonal health.

3. **CHOOSE THE RIGHT SWEETS.** Decrease the amount of sugar you take in as much as possible, including fruits high in sugar, such as mangoes and grapes.

4. **AVOID JUNK FOOD.** It's just empty calories.

5. **DRINK PLENTY OF FILTERED OR SPRING WATER.** Avoid chronic dehydration, as it may prolong healing.

6. **SLEEP.** At least seven hours a night. Lack of sleep can cause a decline in your health and recovery.

7. **TAKE YOUR SUPPLEMENTS.** A multivitamin/mineral complex from whole food source is recommended over the synthetic kind. Vitamin D supplementation is a must to decrease infections and promote healthy bone. Omega-3 supplements promote cellular flexibility, and decrease inflammation. For specific personalized recommendations, see a health practitioner well trained in supplementation.

8. **EXERCISE.** Movement is important for circulation.

9. **MEDITATION.** Five minutes a day is a good start.

10. **EXPLORE.** Energy medicine is here to stay and is becoming more popular. Look into acquiring a home device for healing and balancing your energetic field.

By bringing natural ways to repair, rebuild, and renew into your life, you will not only feel better, look better, and move better, but you will heal better.

Remember: The ability to heal well means maintaining good health throughout your lifetime. My book is a comprehensive resource, so anytime you feel yourself straying from your health and healing journey, simply open these pages and reread the chapter that speaks to you. Whether you need to revisit the chapter on food; light and energy; mediation, guided imagery, and sleep; oxygen; plants, herbs, and teas; supplements; or water, you will find vital information on natural health and healing.

I am grateful for your trust in allowing me to bring you the latest nutritional news to optimize your health and healing. Thank you for joining me on this journey.

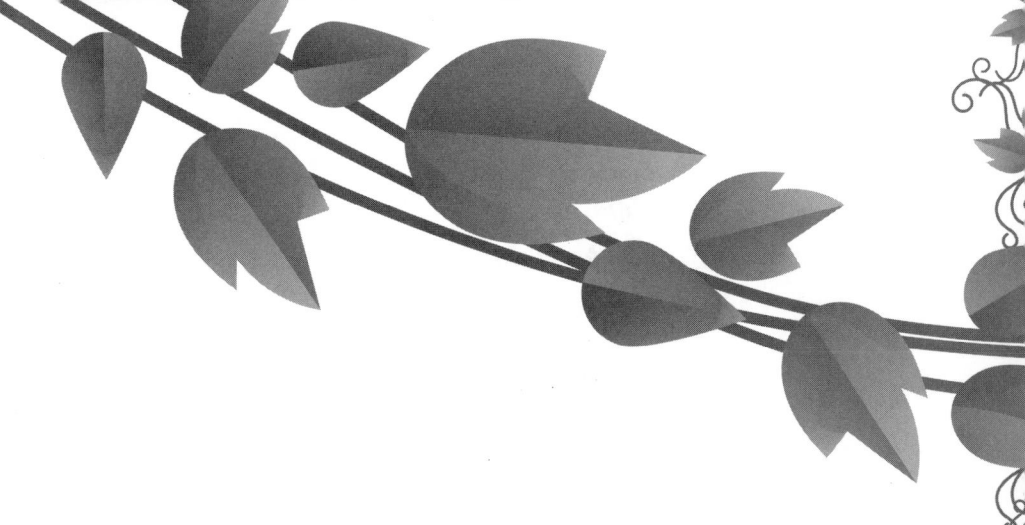

RECIPES FOR HEALING

Let's face it, who wants to cook when they've just had surgery? These recipes require minimal preparation and cleanup so you can get the rest necessary for healing. I picked these recipes because they are low in acidity, which means there will be little, if any, burning sensation for patients using them after oral surgery. However, everyone can enjoy these recipes.

These recipes require a good blender, such as a Blendtec or Vitamix brand, especially for those recipes with nuts in order to make sure they are blended well. These brands of blenders can also heat up the soups while blending, eliminating the additional step of heating the soup afterward.

I intentionally left out fruits with little seeds, such as strawberries, blueberries, and goji berries. These are to be avoided in the first week after oral surgery, as they can get lodged under the mucosa and possibly cause an infection.

If you don't have one of the ingredients listed, such as maca, tocotrienol, or phytoplankton, you may purchase them at your local natural food store or online at Amazon.com.

I included a number of soup recipes because, simply put, I love soups. My mom used to make me soup whenever I was sick and, growing up, we had soup every day. I still crave a nice, warm bowl soup to give me that sense of comfort.

I am by no means suggesting that a person recovering from surgery should only consume liquids while they are healing. In fact, it is best not to consume overly sugary smoothies while healing as sugar, even if it's natural, can cause inflammation.

I have included both savory and sweet blended recipes for those times when you need a quick, delicious, and nutritious meal. Please try both the savory and sweet recipes to create a balance of flavors throughout your healing.

In great health,

Dr. Sanda

SOUPS

Curried Pumpkin Soup

This soup is rich in vitamin A which is important for healing the skin and the oral cavity.

1 tablespoon olive oil or avocado oil

¼ cup chopped onion

2 tablespoons curry powder

16 oz pumpkin—frozen or pureed

2 cups organic vegetable broth

14 oz coconut/almond milk

Pinch of salt

In a large pot, heat the oil over a medium/low heat. Add the onions with a pinch of salt and cook for three to five minutes. Add the curry powder, pumpkin puree, and the broth and let simmer for ten minutes. Add salt and pepper to taste. Puree the soup in a blender and add the coconut/almond milk.

Butternut Squash Soup

2 cups diced butternut squash

¼ cup hemp seeds

½ teaspoon chopped rosemary

1 small chopped tomato

1 garlic clove

1 tablespoon lemon juice

3 tablespoons extra virgin avocado oil

2 cups warm water

Salt and pepper to taste

Blend all ingredients until smooth.

....

Savory Blended Soup (no cooking necessary)

2 cups spring water

½ cup chopped red bell pepper

½ cup chopped cucumber

¼ cup chopped celery

3 or 4 sprigs parsley

2 or 3 stalks of kale

¼ onion

1 tablespoon spirulina or blue-green algae

Salt to taste

Blend all ingredients until smooth.

....

Avocado-Cucumber Soup (no cooking necessary)

1 small ripe avocado

1 cucumber

1 handful of spinach - fresh or frozen

1 garlic clove

½ cup water

1 tablespoon extra-virgin olive oil

1 tablespoon lemon juice

1 tablespoon fresh-chopped dill or cilantro

Blend all ingredients until smooth.

....

Miso Zucchini Soup

1 medium zucchini, chopped

1 celery stalk, chopped

1 clove garlic

½ ripe avocado

1 tablespoon extra-virgin olive oil

¾ cup water

1 tablespoon lemon juice

1 tablespoon miso paste

1 tablespoon fresh dill

1 teaspoon nutritional yeast

Salt and pepper to taste

Blend all ingredients until smooth.

....

SMOOTHIES

Energy Smoothie

2 cups coconut milk

1 scoop vanilla protein powder

1 tablespoon coconut oil

1 teaspoon HealthForce Vitamineral Green

1 teaspoon Maca powder

1 teaspoon bee pollen

1 teaspoon vanilla extract or fresh vanilla bean

1 teaspoon raw honey

Blend all ingredients until smooth.

Chocolate-Vanilla Smoothie

2 cups water or any nut milk

1 tablespoon cacao, preferably raw and fair trade

1 banana

2 tablespoons protein powder – vegan or whey

½ teaspoon cinnamon

½ teaspoon Maca

1 tablespoon coconut butter or oil

1 tablespoon honey, agave, or xylitol (must be dissolved in ½ cup of water before adding)

1 tablespoon hemp seeds

1 tablespoon tocotrienols (vitamin E source)

1 tablespoon natural vanilla extract

2 tablespoons aloe vera juice or fresh aloe

Pinch salt

Blend all ingredients until smooth.

Mango Delight

2 cups water or almond milk

1 mango, peeled and cubed

1 teaspoon lime juice

½ cup cashews

1 tablespoon tocotrienol

Blend all ingredients until smooth.

....

Papaya and Banana Smoothie

1 Hawaiian papaya

½ lime peeled

1 banana

1 cup coconut water

10 drops silica

½ cup vanilla protein—vegan or whey

2 capfuls Morningstar minerals

Blend all ingredients until smooth.

....

Watermelon-Mint Smoothie (can substitute cantaloupe)

2 cups cubed watermelon or cantaloupe

1 cup coconut water

5-6 fresh mint leaves

1 tablespoon tocotrienols

1 teaspoon lime juice

2 full droppers marine phytoplankton

2 ounces Morningstar Minerals Energy Boost

Blend all ingredients until smooth.

Peanut Butter and Jelly Smoothie

2 cups almond milk

2 tablespoons organic peanut butter

2 tablespoons cherry preserves

1 banana

1 tablespoon tocotrienols

Blend all ingredients until smooth.

....

Chocolate Pudding

2 ripe avocadoes

1 tablespoon raw cacao powder

½ teaspoon vanilla

2 tablespoon agave nectar or raw honey

Salt to taste

Cinnamon to taste

Blend all ingredients until smooth. Refrigerate or freeze any leftovers.

....

Grape Yogurt Smoothie

1 cup seedless grapes

1 cup yogurt

1 tablespoon agave nectar

1 tablespoon lemon juice

Blend all ingredients until smooth.

Coconut-Peach Cream

Flesh from 2 young coconuts

2 ripe peaches

2 tablespoons hemp seeds

1 teaspoon vanilla extract

1 tablespoon tocontrienols

1 tablespoon lucuma powder

1 tablespoon coconut oil

½ cup coconut water

Blend all ingredients until smooth.

JUICING

Juicing is a great way to nourish and detoxify. The biggest problem that I see with most of my patients who are juicing is that they drink juices that are too sweet. For example, grape juice is not a healthy juice, especially for diabetics, because of its high-glycemic index. Grapes, beets, carrots, and apples, for example, have a high sugar concentration and, even though it is natural sugar, it is not healthy to raise blood sugar levels so fast. These fruits and vegetables are better to be eaten whole because the fiber prevents the fast absorption of sugar from the intestines, which is much healthier. When juicing, I advise you to mix 30 to 40 percent fruits and colored vegetables with 60 to 70 percent green vegetables. Colored vegetables, such as bell pepper, carrots, and beets have more sugar, whereas green vegetables, such as kale, cucumber, celery, and parsley have a low-glycemic index.

I don't juice as a routine, because I believe fruits and vegetables are meant to be eaten whole. Juices are great for recovery and healing and I encourage you to try some of the recipes below.

Anti-Inflammatory Juice

Celery has at least a dozen antioxidants, but most importantly, its phytonutrients have been shown to reduce inflammation in the digestive tract and blood vessels.

3 stalks celery

1 medium cucumber

1 orange peeled

½ apple with seeds

½ bunch parsley (optional)

Sulphur-rich Juice

1 bunch kale

1 medium cucumber

1 bunch arugula

1 cup broccoli

1 orange

1 cup coconut water

Veggie Juice

1 carrot

2 celery stalks

½ cup red cabbage

1 red pepper

½ cucumber

1 bunch parsley

1 red radish

1 teaspoon lemon juice

Green Juice

3 kale or Swiss chard leaves

2 celery stalks

1 cucumber

½ bunch cilantro

½ cup water

Sea salt to taste

Essential Juice

2 celery stalks

2 apples

1 cup spinach

1 cup kale

2 tablespoons of E3Live (E3Live contains vitamin B12, essential fatty acids, and twenty-two amino acids)

Savory Celery Almond Drink

1 bunch celery juiced to make 1 cup juice

1 cucumber juiced

1 cup almond milk

1 clove garlic

1 teaspoon sea salt

2 tablespoons lemon juice

REFERENCES

••

Chapter 1

1. "Adult Obesity Facts," Centers for Disease Control and Prevention, last modified August 29, 2017, https://www.cdc.gov/obesity/data/adult.html.

2. Elizabeth Motyka, M. Nathaniel Mead, and Tom Motyka, *The Rapid Recovery Handbook: Your Complete Guide to Faster Healing After Surgery* (William Morrow Paperbacks, 2016).

3. Liu Z, Li N, and Neu J, "Tight junctions, leaky intestines, and pediatric diseases," *Acta Paediatr* 94, no. 4 (April 2005): 386–93.

4. Tainya C. Clarke, Tina Norris, and Jeannine S. Schiller, "Early Release of Selected Estimates Based on Data From the 2016 National Health Interview Survey," National Center for Health Statistics, last modified May 2017, http://www.cdc.gov/nchs/nhis.htm.

5. Tammy Carullo, "Part 6: Nutrition: More than just the basic four!" *RDH*, accessed May 9, 2017, http://www.rdhmag.com/articles/print/volume-22/issue-1/feature/part-6-nutrition-more-than-just-the-basic-four.html.

6. "Tobacco-Related Mortality," Centers for Disease Control and Prevention, last modified December 1, 2016, https://www.

cdc.gov/tobacco/data_statistics/fact_sheets/health_effects/
tobacco_related_mortality/.

Chapter 2

1. Amir Azarpazhooh, Herenia P. Lawrence, and Prakeshkumar S. Shah, "Xylitol for preventing acute otitis media in children up to 12 years of age," Cochrane Acute Respiratory Infections Group, last modified August 3, 2016, http://onlinelibrary.wiley.com/doi/10.1002/14651858.CD007095.pub3/abstract.

2. Chinsembu, K.C., "Plants and other natural products used in the management of oral infections and improvement of oral health," *Acta tropica* (2016): 1546–18, http://www.sciencedirect.com/science/article/pii/S0001706X1530142X.

3. Elizabeth Walling, "Stop bad breath and body odor with chlorophyll," Natural News, accessed May 8, 2017, http://www.naturalnews.com/032913_bad_breath_chlorophyll.html.

4. MC Fadus et al., "Curcumin: Age-Old Anti-Inflammatory and Anti-Neoplastic Agent," Journal of Traditional Contemporary Medicine 7, no.3 (September 2009): 339–346.

5. Meletis, Chris, "Mitochondria Resuscitation: The Key to Healing Every Disease," Complementary Prescriptions, accessed May 11, 2017, http://www.cpmedical.net/newsletter/mitochondria-resuscitation-the-key-to-healing-every-disease.

6. P. A. S. Theophilis et al., "Effectiveness of *Stevia Rebaudiana* Whole Leaf Extract Against the Various Morphological Forms of *Borrelia Burgdorferi in Vitro*," *Eurpoean Journal of Microbiology & Immunology* 5, no. 4 (December 2015): 268–280.

7. Silva, F., et al., "Coriander (*Coriandrum sativum* L.) essential oil: its antibacterial activity and mode of action evaluated by flow cytometry," *Journal of Medical Microbiology* 60 (October 1, 2011): 1479–1486, http://jmm.microbiologyresearch.org/content/journal/jmm/10.1099/jmm.0.034157-0.

8. Southward, K., "A hypothetical role for vitamin K2 in the endocrine and exocrine aspects of dental caries," *Medical Hypotheses* 84, no. 3 (2015): 276–80.

Chapter 3

1. Azeemi, Samina and S. Raza, "A Critical Analysis of Chromotherapy and Its Scientific Evolution," *Evidence-Based Complementary and Alternative Medicine* 2, no. 4 (2005): 481–488, https://www.ncbi.nlm.nih.gov/pmc/articles/PMC1297510/.

2. Brunelli Roberta , et al., "The effects of 780-nm low-level laser therapy on muscle healing process after cryolesion," *Lasers in Medical Science* 28, no. 1 (February 2013): 91–96.

3. B Lipton. *The Biology of Belief*, (Hay House, 2004).

4. Mao, H.S., M. Yao, and Y. Fang, "Advancement in the research of effect of low level laser therapy on wound healing," *Zhonghua Shao Shang Za Zhi (Chinese Journal of Burns)* 28, no. 6 (December 2012): 462–5, https://www.ncbi.nlm.nih.gov/pubmed/23327917.

5. Martin, D.P., "Improvement in fibromyalgia symptoms with acupuncture: results of a randomized controlled trial." Mayo Clinic Proceedings 81, no. 6 (June 2006): 749–57.

6. Mayo Clinic. "Which alternative cancer treatments are worth trying?" Accessed May 10, 2017. http://www.mayoclinic.org/diseases-conditions/cancer/in-depth/cancer-treatment/art-20047246?pg=2.

7. McMillen, Matt, "Acupuncture Goes Mainstream," WebMD, accessed May 10, 2017, http://www.webmd.com/balance/features/acupuncture-goes-mainstream#1.

8. Mercola, Joseph, "Are You Making These Sunshine Mistakes?" Mercola, September 29, 2012, accessed March 1, 2017, http://articles.mercola.com/sites/articles/archive/2012/09/29/sun-exposure-vitamin-d-production-benefits.aspx.

9. Mercola, Joseph, "Caution: Wearing These Can Sabotage Your Health," interview with James Oschman, Mercola, April 29, 2012, http://articles.mercola.com/sites/articles/archive/2012/04/29/james-oschman-on-earthing.aspx.

10. Ober, Clinton, et al., *Earthing: The Most Important Health Discovery Ever!* 2nd ed. Basic Health Publications, 2014.

11. Samina, T., Yousuf Azeemi, and S. Mohsin Raza, "A Critical Analysis of Chromotherapy and Its Scientific Evolution." *Evidence-Based Complementary and Alternative Medicine* 2, no. 4 (December 2005): 481–488. https://www.ncbi.nlm.nih.gov/pmc/articles/PMC1297510/.

12. "Testing for vitamin D." Accessed May 10, 2017. https://www.vitamindcouncil.org/about-vitamin-d/testing-for-vitamin-d/.

13. Tuner, Jan, and Lars Hode, *The Laser Therapy Handbook.* Sweden: Prima Books, 2004.

Chapter 4

1. Abler, Alice, "The Vital role of sleep in good health." *Price-Pottenger Journal* 38, no. 3 (October 13, 2014): 4-12. https://price-pottenger.org/journals/vital-role-sleep-good-health.

2. Carr, Kris, *Crazy Sexy Cancer Survivor: More Rebellion And Fire For Your Healing Journey.* Lanham: Rowman & Littlefield Publishers, 2008.

3. Chang, K., et al., "Chronic pain management: nonpharmacological therapies for chronic pain." *FP Essentials* 432 (May 2015): 21-6.

4. Del Casale, A., et al., "Pain perception and hypnosis: findings from recent functional neuroimaging studies." *International Journal of Clinical and Experimental Hypnosis* 63, no. 2 (2015): 144-70.

5. Enqvist, B. and K. Fischer, "Preoperative hypnotic techniques reduce consumption of analgesics after surgical removal of third mandibular

molars: a brief communication." *International Journal of Clinical and Experimental Hypnosis* 45, no. 2 (April 1997): 102-8.

6. Enqvist B, et al., "Preoperative hypnosis reduces postoperative vomiting after surgery of the breasts. A prospective, randomized and blinded study." *Acta Anaesthesiologica Scandinavica* 41, no. 8 (September 1997): 1028-32.

7. Fife, Caroline, et al., "An Update on the Appropriate Role for Hyperbaric Oxygen: Indications and Evidence." *Plastic and Reconstructive Surgery* 138, no. 3 (September 2016): 107S–116S. https://www.ncbi.nlm.nih.gov/pmc/articles/PMC4996355/.

8. Ginandes, C, et al., "Can medical hypnosis accelerate post-surgical wound healing? Results of a clinical trial." *American Journal of Clinical Hypnosis* 45, no. 4 (April 2003): 333-51.

9. Ginandes, C. and D. Rosenthal, "Using hypnosis to accelerate the healing of bone fractures: a randomized controlled pilot study." *Alternative Therapies, Health and Medicine* 5, no. 2 (March 1999): 67-75.

10. Gomez-Pinilla, F., et al., "The influence of exercise on cognitive abilities." Comprehensive Physiology 3, no. 1 (January 2013): 403-428. https://www.ncbi.nlm.nih.gov/pmc/articles/PMC3951958/.

11. Holroyd J, "Hypnosis treatment of clinical pain: understanding why hypnosis is useful." International Journal of Clinical and Experimental Hypnosis 44, no. 1 (January 1996): 33-51.

12. Huddleston, Peggy, *Prepare for surgery, heal faster.* 5th ed. Cambridge: Angel River Press, 2013.

13. Jennum P, et al. "Social consequences of sleep disordered breathing on patients and their partners: a controlled national study" *European Respiratory Journal* 43, no. 1 (January 2014): 134-144.

14. Jensen, M. and D. Patterson, "Hypnotic treatment of chronic pain." *Journal of Behavioral Medicine* 29, no. 1 (February 2006): 95-124.

15. Kabat-Zinn, Jon. *Full Catastrophe Living: Using the Wisdom of Your Body and Mind to Face Stress, Pain, and Illness.* New York: Bantam Books, 2013.

16. Kabat-Zinn, Jon and Richard Davidson, *The Mind's Own Physician: A Scientific Dialogue with the Dalai Lama on the Healing Power of Meditation.* Oakland: New Harbinger, 2012.

17. Kravitx, Kathy, "Hypnosis for the Management of Anticipatory Nausea and Vomiting." *Journal of the Advanced Practitioner in Oncology* 6, no. 3 (May-June 2015): 225–229. https://www.ncbi.nlm.nih.gov/pmc/articles/PMC4625628/.

18. Lazar, S., et al., "Meditation experience is associated with increased cortical thickness." *NeuroReport* 16, no. 17 (November 28, 2005): 1893-97. https://www.ncbi.nlm.nih.gov/pmc/articles/PMC1361002/.

19. Little, P. "Randomised controlled trial of Alexander technique lessons, exercise, and massage (ATEAM) for chronic and recurrent back pain." *BMJ* 337 (August 19, 2008).

20. National Sleep Foundation. "Let sleep work for you." Accessed March 5, 2018. https://sleepfoundation.org/how-sleep-works/how-much-sleep-do-we-really-need.

21. McCabe, Ed, *Flood Your Body with Oxygen.* Spring Lake: Breath of God Ministries, 2004.

22. Patterson, D. and M. Jensen. "Hypnosis and clinical pain." *Psychological Bulletin* 129, no. 4 (July 2003): 495-521.

23. Roehrs, T., et al. "Sleep loss and REM sleep loss are hyperalgesic." *Sleep* 29, no. 2 (February 2006): 145-151.

24. Rossignol, DA. "Hyperbaric oxygen treatment in autism spectrum disorders." *Medical Gas Research* 2, no. 16 (2012). https://www.ncbi.nlm.nih.gov/pmc/articles/PMC3472266/.

25. Sharma, S., et al. "Sleep and metabolism: an overview." *International Journal of Endocrinology* (2010).

26. International Agency for Research on Cancer. "Shiftwork." *IARC Monographs on the Evaluation of Carcinogenic Risks to Humans* 98, (2010). monographs.iarc.fr/ENG/Monographs.

27. Sourabh, Bhutani and Guruswamy Vishwanath. "Hyperbaric oxygen and wound healing." Indian Journal of Plastic Surgery 45, no. 2 (May-August 2012): 316–324. https://www.ncbi.nlm.nih.gov/pmc/articles/PMC3495382/.

28. American Lung Association. "Supplemental Oxygen." Accessed May 10, 2017. http://www.lung.org/lung-health-and-diseases/lung-disease-lookup/copd/diagnosing-and-treating/supplemental-oxygen.html.

29. Wobst, A. "Hypnosis and surgery: past, present, and future." *Anesthesia & Analgesia* 104, no. 5 (May 2007): 1199-208.

Chapter 5

1. Bocci, V., et al. "The ozone paradox: ozone is a strong oxidant as well as a medical drug." *Medicinal Research Reviews* 29, no. 4 (2009): 646-682.

2. Gajendrareddy. P., et al. "Hyperbaric oxygen therapy ameliorates stress-impaired dermal wound healing." *Brain, Behavior, and Immunity* 19, no. 3 (2005): 217-222.

3. Gordillo, G. and C. Sen. "Evidence-based recommendations for the use of topical oxygen therapy in the treatment of lower extremity wounds." *The International Journal of Lower Extremity Wounds* 8, no. 2 (2009): 105-111.

4. Kim, H., et al. "Therapeutic effects of topical application of ozone on acute cutaneous wound healing." *Journal of Korean Medical Science* 24, no. 3 (2009): 368–374.

5. McCabe, Ed. *Flood Your Body with Oxygen*. Spring Lake: Breath of God Ministries, 2004.

6.   Menéndez, S., L. Falcón, and Y. Maqueira. "Therapeutic efficacy of topical OLEOZON® in patients suffering from onychomycosis." *Mycoses* 54, no. 5 (September 2011): 272-7.

7.   Plafki, C. et al. "Complications and side effects of hyperbaric oxygen therapy." Aviation, Space, and Environmental Medicine 71, no. 2 (February 2000): 119-24. http://www.ncbi.nlm.nih.gov/pubmed/10685584.

8.   Rappolt, R. "The ozone generator." *Clinical Toxicology* 5, no. 3 (1972): 419-425.

9.   Stoker, G. "The surgical use of ozone." *The Lancet* 188, no. 4860 (1916): 712.

10. The University of Maryland Medical Center. "Herbal medicine." Accessed May 10, 2017. http://www.umm.edu/altmed/articles/herbal-medicine-000351.htm.

11. Travagli, V. et. al. "Ozone and Ozonated Oils in Skin Diseases: A Review." *Mediators of Inflammation* (2010).

12. Travagli, V., I. Zanardi, and V. Bocci. "Topical applications of ozone and ozonated oils as anti-infective agents: an insight into the patent claims." *Recent Patents on Anti-Infective Drug Discovery* 4, no. 2 (2009): 130-142.

13. Valacchi, G. et al., "Evaluation of ozonated sesame oil effect in wound healing using the SKH1 mice as a model." *Proceeding of the 7th World Meeting on Pharmaceutics, Biopharmaceutics and Pharmaceutical Technology* (2010).

Chapter 6

14. Aroma Tools. *Modern Essentials: A Contemporary Guide to the Therapeutic use of Essential Oils.* Aroma Tools, 2009.

15. Jones, Elizabeth. *Awaken to Healing Fragrance: The power of essential oil therapy* Berkeley: North Atlantic Books, 2010.

16. Long, Josh. "FDA GMP Inspectors Cite 70% of Dietary Supplement Firms." accessed May 10, 2017. https://www.naturalproductsinsider. com/news/2013/05/fda-gmp-inspectors-cite-70-of-dietary-supplement.aspx.

17. Mayo Clinic. *Book of Alternative Medicine: The new approach to using the best of natural therapies and conventional medicine.* New York: Time Inc., 2007.

18. Mercola, Joseph and Rachael Droege. "Top Five Essential Oils for Your Health." Last modified March 13, 2004. http://articles.mercola. com/sites/articles/archive/2004/03/13/essential-oils.aspx.

19. *The Herb Companion*

20. The University of Maryland Medical Center. "Herbal Medicine." Accessed March 5, 2018. http://www.umm.edu/altmed/articles/ herbal-medicine-000351.htm.

Chapter 7

1. Anahad O'Connor. "New York Attorney General Targets Supplements at Major Retailers." *The New York Times*. Last modified February 3, 2015. https://well.blogs.nytimes.com/2015/02/03/ new-york-attorney-general-targets-supplements-at-major-retailers/.

2. Centers for Disease Control and Prevention. "Antibiotic/ Antimicrobial Resistance." Accessed May 11, 2017. https://www.cdc. gov/drugresistance/index.html.

3. Donaldson, M. and R. Touger-Decker. "Dietary supplement interactions with medications used commonly in dentistry." *The Journal of the American Dental Association* 144, no. 7 (2013): 787-94.

4. "Exercise caution when combining medications. Many over-the-counter medications and dietary supplements can have negative interactions with your prescription drugs," *The Cleveland Clinic Heart Advisor* 12, no. 5 (2009): 6.

5.   Howell, Edward. *Food Enzymes for Health & Longevity*. (Lotus Press, 1994).

6.   Lee, A.H. et al. "The incidence of potential interactions between dietary supplements and prescription medications in cancer patients at a Veterans Administration Hospital." *American Journal of Clinical Oncology* 29, no. 2 (2006): 178-82.

7.   Mangin, M. et al. "Inflammation and vitamin D: the infection connection." *Inflammation Research* 63, no. 10 (2014): 803–819.

8.   National Institutes of Health State-of-the-Science. "National Institutes of Health State-of-the-Science Conference Statement: multivitamin/ mineral supplements and chronic disease prevention." *American Journal of Clinical Nutrition* 85, no. 1 (2007): 257S-64S.

9.   O'Connor, Anahad. "New York Attorney General Targets Supplements at Major Retailers." February 3, 2015. Accessed May 10, 2017. https:// well.blogs.nytimes.com/2015/02/03/new-york-attorney-general-targets-supplements-at-major-retailers/?_r=0.

10. Price, Weston. "Nutrition and Physical Degeneration." Price Pottenger, 2009.

11. Schmidt, Sarah. "Tea Sales on an Upward Trend in the U.S." Market Research. Accessed May 10, 2017. http://blog.marketresearch.com/ tea-sales-on-an-upward-trend.

12. Sood, A. et al. "Potential for interactions between dietary supplements and prescription medications." *The American Journal of Medicine* 121, no. 3 (2008): 207-11.

13. Throckmorton, Douglas. "Re-scheduling prescription hydrocodone combination drug products: An important step toward controlling misuse and abuse." U.S. Food & Drug Administration. Accessed May 10, 2017. https://blogs.fda.gov/fdavoice/index.php/2014/10/ re-scheduling-prescription-hydrocodone-combination-drug-products-an-important-step-toward-controlling-misuse-and-abuse/.

14. Zupancic, K. et al. "Influence of Oral Probiotic Streptococcus salivarius K12 on Ear and Oral Cavity Health in Humans: Systematic Review." *Probiotics and Antimicrobial Proteins* (2017).

Chapter 8

1. Batmanghelidj, F. *You're not sick, you're thirsty! Water for Health, for Healing, for Life.* Grand Central Life & Style, 2003.

2. Batmanghelidj, F. *Your Body's Many Cries for Water.* Grand Central Life & Style, 1992.

3. Blackburn, G. "Does oxygenated water offer any special health benefits?" *Health News* 10, no. 1 (January 2004): 16.

4. Cotter, J., et al., "Are we being drowned in hydration advice? Thirsty for more?" *Extreme Physiology & Medicine* (October 29, 2014): 3-18. doi: 10.1186/2046-7648-3-18. eCollection 2014. Review.

5. Efimenko NV, Kalslnova AS. "The spa-and-health resort-based rehabilitation of the patients presenting with frequently recurring erosive and ulcerative lesions in the oesophagus, stomach, and duodenum in the phase of subsiding exacerbation." *Vopr Kurortol Fizioter Lech Fiz Kult* no. 4 (July-August 2014): 17-21.

6. Gruber R., S. Axmann, and M. Schoenberg. "The influence of oxygenated water on the immune status, liver enzymes, and the generation of oxygen radicals: a prospective, randomised, blinded clinical study." *Clinical Nutrition* 24, no. 3 (June 2005): 407-14.

7. Jequier, E. and F. Constant. "Water as an essential nutrient: the physiological basis of hydration." *European Journal of Clinical Nutrition* 64 (2010): 115-23.

8. Kavouras, S. "Assessing hydration status." *Current Opinion in Clinical Nutrition and Metabolic Care* 5, no. 5 (September 2002): 519-24.

9. Marcos, A. et al. "Physical activity, hydration and health." *Nutricion hospitalaria* 29, no. 6 (June 1, 2014): 1224-39. doi: 10.3305/nh.2014.29.6.7624.

10. Millard-Stafford, M. "Thirst and hydration status in everyday life." *Nutrition Reviews* 70 (2012): S147-51.

11. Murray, B. "Hydration and physical performance." *Journal of the American College of Nutritio* 26, no. 5 (October 2007): 542S-548S.

12. Nagayoshi, M., et al. "Antimicrobial effect of ozonated water on bacteria invading dentinal tubules." *Journal of Endodontics* 30, no. 11 (November 2004): 778-81.

13. Nogales, C., et al. "Ozone therapy in medicine and dentistry." *Journal of Contemporary Dental Practice* 9, no. 4 (May 1, 2008): 75-84.

14. Popkin, B., K. D'Anci, and I. Rosenberg. "Water, hydration, and health." *Nutrition Reviews* 68 (2010): 439-58.

15. Riebl, S. "The Hydration Equation: Update on Water Balance and Cognitive Performance." *ACSM'S Health & Fitness Journal* 17, no. 6 (November 2013): 21-28.

16. Rosinger, A. and S. Tanner. "Water from fruit or the river? Examining hydration strategies and gastrointestinal illness among Tsimane' adults in the Bolivian Amazon." *Public Health Nutrition* (October 7, 2014): 1-11.

17. Schoenberg, M., et al. "The generation of oxygen radicals after drinking of oxygenated water." *European Journal of Medical Research* 7, no. 3 (March 28, 2002): 109-16.

18. Stübinger, S., R. Sader, and A. Filippi. "The use of ozone in dentistry and maxillofacial surgery: a review." *Quintessence International* 37, no. 5 (May 2006): 353-9.

19. Taylor, Jeffrey. "Ozonated Water, Also known as Ozone Water, Ozo-Water." http://www.oxygenhealingtherapies.com/ozonated_water.html.

20. Valtin, H. " 'Drink at least eight glasses of water a day.' Really? Is there scientific evidence for '8 x 8'?" *American Journal of Physiology. Regulatory, Integrative and Comparative Physiology* 283, no. 5 (November 2002): R993-1004.

21. Wolf, R., et al., "Nutrition and water: drinking eight glasses of water a day ensures proper skin hydration-myth or reality?" *Clinics in Dermatology* 28, no. 4 (July-August 2010): 380-3. doi: 10.1016/j.clindermatol.2010.03.022.

OUR SERVICES

....

Beverly Hills Dental Health and Wellness takes an entirely different approach to dentistry. Our team of highly qualified professionals know that your mouth is the gateway to overall health. We have the superior training and experience to implement a foundation of dental care that improves your wellness, quality of life ... as well as your smile! As our patient, you are assured the healthy and beautiful result you desire and deserve, as we understand the connection between your mouth and body, treating it as one.

The Beverly Hills Dental Health and Wellness team includes:

A periodontist focused on tissues and structures surrounding teeth.	**A nutritionist with unique insight into optimum wellness and recovery.**
A regenerative endodontist who specializes in maintaining teeth through treatment of the vital inner structure.	**A prosthodontist for full-mouth rehabilitations.**
A restorative dentist who uses healthy biocompatible materials and techniques for general procedures, such as safe amalgam fillings and removal.	**A chiropractor whose treatment skills complement whole-health dentistry.**

The team at Beverly Hills Dental Health and Wellness is dedicated to the practice of biological dentistry. Together, these individuals form an unparalleled lineup of like-minded professionals, committed to a higher level of oral healthcare, providing services such as:

A customized health and wellness plan	Ceramic dental implants	Full mouth restoration
Laser gum disease treatment and inflammation management	Biocompatible restorations and fillings	Vital pulp therapy—to avoid needing a root canal
Mercury-free fillings	Non-metal, biocompatible crowns and bridges Pulp revascularization—stem cell therapy	TMJ and sleep apnea appliances
Treatment to minimize tooth sensitivity with ozone, laser, and homeopathic techniques		

Dentistry isn't about teeth; it's about people. It's about you, your health, and your ability to live life to the fullest. Seemingly minor oral problems can signify nutritional deficiencies, medical conditions, and other health concerns. Digestion begins in the mouth. Improving oral health can help improve overall physical health; the reverse is also true. There is an unending list of reasons that oral wellness is important. Your mouth is the gateway to your health.

  FOLLOW US!

Instagram: @drsanda
https://www.instagram.com/drsanda/

Youtube: @askdrsanda
https://www.youtube.com/user/AskDrSanda/

Twitter: @drsanda
https://www.twitter.com/drsanda

Facebook: @askdrsanda
http://facebook.com/askdrsanda

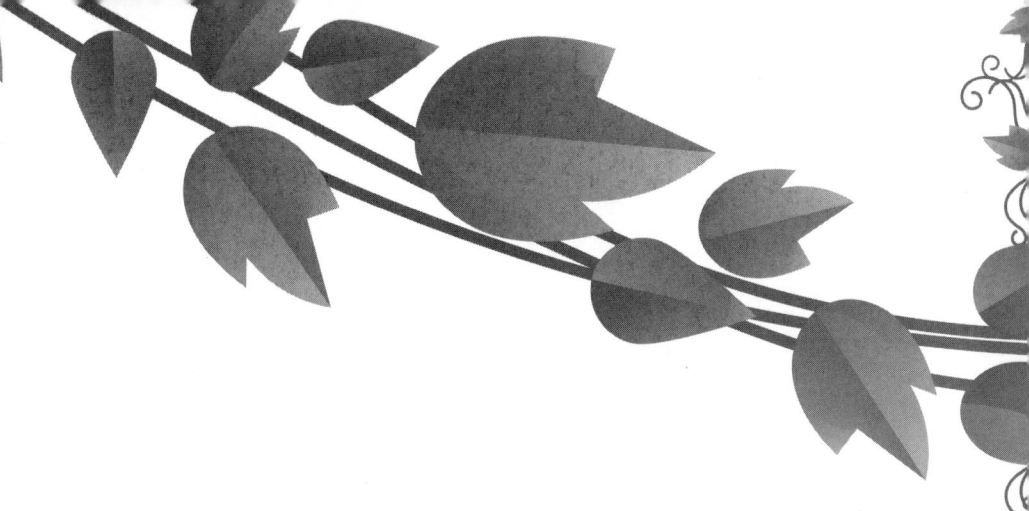

ABOUT THE AUTHOR

Sanda Moldovan, D.D.S., the founder of Beverly Hills Dental Health and Wellness, is an award-winning periodontist, and world-renowned oral health and wellness expert. The developer of the Orasana natural oral product line, she continues to make significant advancements in achieving greater personal oral health care with probiotic supplements and home dental care products for adults and children's teeth and gums. In addition to being double board-certified in periodontics and nutrition, she is recognized as a leading authority on natural and safe anti-aging solutions. She tirelessly promotes non-narcotic alternatives for healing.

Warmly known as Dr. Sanda, her award-winning expertise in biological dentistry has enabled countless patients to learn how to bridge the gap between their mouths and their bodies. As one of the nation's leading advocates for nutritional and homeopathic support for oral health and healing, she frequently appears on the Emmy-winning television show, "The Doctors," as well as guest spots on "Inside Edition," and NBC News. Her patients are from all walks of life. Working mothers, police officers, educators, CEO's, athletes, and Hollywood celebrities; they all share the common desire to live and long and healthier life.

The YouTube channel Ask Dr. Sanda champions education and public awareness for making better nutrition choices and oral health disciplines. She has authored articles for numerous scientific journals and contributed to major mainstream publications such as *Reader's Digest, Livestrong, Prevention, Men's Health, The Dallas Morning News, The Huffington Post, Life Extension* and *Well Being Journal.*

Dr. Sanda Moldovan is a graduate of the Ohio State University School of Dentistry, with post-graduate training from the University of California, Los Angeles, where she received her master's degree in Oral Biology. She is a faculty member at Global Institute of Dental Education (gIDE). She is a member of the Institute of Functional Medicine, American College of Nutrition, Academy of Anti-Aging Medicine and National Speakers Association, and is a Diplomate of the American Academy of Periodontology.

Dr. Sanda sees patients at her institute in Beverly Hills, California and in Manhattan, New York. She is a philanthropist, committed to helping others transform their health and lives. Her all women team of dental professionals, also known as 'Smile Fairies,' regularly donate dental services to those less fortunate.